Statistics at Square Two

Statistics at Square Two

Understanding Modern Statistical Application in Medicine

Michael J. Campbell
Emeritus Professor of Medical Statistics
University of Sheffield
Sheffield, UK

Richard M. Jacques
Senior Lecture in Medical Statistics
University of Sheffield
Sheffield, UK

Third Edition

WILEY Blackwell

This edition first published 2023

Edition History
©1e, 2001 by BMJ Books
©2e, 2006 by M. J. Campbell

Registered Offices
John Wiley & Sons, Inc., 111 River Street, Hoboken, NJ 07030, USA
John Wiley & Sons Ltd, The Atrium, Southern Gate, Chichester, West Sussex, PO19 8SQ, UK

For details of our global editorial offices, customer services, and more information about Wiley products visit us at www.wiley.com.

Wiley also publishes its books in a variety of electronic formats and by print-on-demand. Some content that appears in standard print versions of this book may not be available in other formats.

Library of Congress Cataloging-in-Publication Data
Names: Campbell, Michael J., 1950- author. | Jacques, Richard M., author.
Title: Statistics at square two : understanding modern statistical applications in medicine / Michael J. Campbell, Emeritus Professor of Medical Statistics, University of Sheffield, Sheffield, UK, Richard M. Jacques, Senior Lecturer in Medical Statistics, University of Sheffield, Sheffield, UK.
Description: Third edition. | Hoboken : John Wiley & Sons, [2023] | Includes bibliographical references and index.
Identifiers: LCCN 2022057672 (print) | LCCN 2022057673 (ebook) | ISBN 9781119401360 (paperback) | ISBN 9781119401377 (pdf) | ISBN 9781119401391 (epub) | ISBN 9781119401407 (ebook)
Subjects: LCSH: Medical statistics--Data processing. | Medical statistics--Computer programs.
Classification: LCC RA409.5 .C36 2023 (print) | LCC RA409.5 (ebook) | DDC 610.2/1--dc23/eng/20221214
LC record available at https://lccn.loc.gov/2022057672
LC ebook record available at https://lccn.loc.gov/2022057673

Cover Image: © Somatuscani/iStock/Getty Images
Cover Design: Wiley

Set in 9.5/12.5pt STIXTwoText by Integra Software Services Pvt. Ltd, Pondicherry, India
Printed and bound by CPI Group (UK) Ltd, Croydon CR0 4YY
C9781119401360_010223

Contents

Preface *xi*

1 **Models, Tests and Data** *1*
1.1 Types of Data *1*
1.2 Confounding, Mediation and Effect Modification *2*
1.3 Causal Inference *3*
1.4 Statistical Models *5*
1.5 Results of Fitting Models *6*
1.6 Significance Tests *7*
1.7 Confidence Intervals *8*
1.8 Statistical Tests Using Models *8*
1.9 Many Variables *9*
1.10 Model Fitting and Analysis: Exploratory and Confirmatory Analyses *10*
1.11 Computer-intensive Methods *11*
1.12 Missing Values *11*
1.13 Bayesian Methods *12*
1.14 Causal Modelling *12*
1.15 Reporting Statistical Results in the Medical Literature *14*
1.16 Reading Statistics in the Medical Literature *14*

2 **Multiple Linear Regression** *17*
2.1 The Model *17*
2.2 Uses of Multiple Regression *18*
2.3 Two Independent Variables *18*
2.3.1 One Continuous and One Binary Independent Variable *19*
2.3.2 Two Continuous Independent Variables *22*
2.3.3 Categorical Independent Variables *22*
2.4 Interpreting a Computer Output *23*
2.4.1 One Continuous Variable *24*
2.4.2 One Continuous Variable and One Binary Independent Variable *25*
2.4.3 One Continuous Variable and One Binary Independent Variable with Their Interaction *26*
2.4.4 Two Independent Variables: Both Continuous *27*
2.4.5 Categorical Independent Variables *29*

2.5 Examples in the Medical Literature *31*
2.5.1 Analysis of Covariance: One Binary and One Continuous Independent Variable *31*
2.5.2 Two Continuous Independent Variables *32*
2.6 Assumptions Underlying the Models *32*
2.7 Model Sensitivity *33*
2.7.1 Residuals, Leverage and Influence *33*
2.7.2 Computer Analysis: Model Checking and Sensitivity *34*
2.8 Stepwise Regression *35*
2.9 Reporting the Results of a Multiple Regression *36*
2.10 Reading about the Results of a Multiple Regression *36*
2.11 Frequently Asked Questions *37*
2.12 Exercises: Reading the Literature *38*

3 Multiple Logistic Regression *41*
3.1 Quick Revision *41*
3.2 The Model *42*
3.2.1 Categorical Covariates *44*
3.3 Model Checking *44*
3.3.1 Lack of Fit *45*
3.3.2 “Extra-binomial” Variation or “Over Dispersion” *45*
3.3.3 The Logistic Transform is Inappropriate *46*
3.4 Uses of Logistic Regression *46*
3.5 Interpreting a Computer Output *47*
3.5.1 One Binary Independent Variable *47*
3.5.2 Two Binary Independent Variables *51*
3.5.3 Two Continuous Independent Variables *53*
3.6 Examples in the Medical Literature *54*
3.6.1 Comment *55*
3.7 Case-control Studies *56*
3.8 Interpreting Computer Output: Unmatched Case-control Study *56*
3.9 Matched Case-control Studies *58*
3.10 Interpreting Computer Output: Matched Case-control Study *58*
3.11 Example of Conditional Logistic Regression in the Medical Literature *60*
3.11.1 Comment *60*
3.12 Alternatives to Logistic Regression *61*
3.13 Reporting the Results of Logistic Regression *61*
3.14 Reading about the Results of Logistic Regression *61*
3.15 Frequently Asked Questions *62*
3.16 Exercise *62*

4 Survival Analysis *65*
4.1 Introduction *65*
4.2 The Model *66*

4.3 Uses of Cox Regression *68*
4.4 Interpreting a Computer Output *68*
4.5 Interpretation of the Model *70*
4.6 Generalisations of the Model *70*
4.6.1 Stratified Models *70*
4.6.2 Time Dependent Covariates *71*
4.6.3 Parametric Survival Models *71*
4.6.4 Competing Risks *71*
4.7 Model Checking *72*
4.8 Reporting the Results of a Survival Analysis *73*
4.9 Reading about the Results of a Survival Analysis *74*
4.10 Example in the Medical Literature *74*
4.10.1 Comment *75*
4.11 Frequently Asked Questions *76*
4.12 Exercises *77*

5 Random Effects Models *79*
5.1 Introduction *79*
5.2 Models for Random Effects *80*
5.3 Random vs Fixed Effects *81*
5.4 Use of Random Effects Models *81*
5.4.1 Cluster Randomised Trials *81*
5.4.2 Repeated Measures *82*
5.4.3 Sample Surveys *83*
5.4.4 Multi-centre Trials *83*
5.5 Ordinary Least Squares at the Group Level *84*
5.6 Interpreting a Computer Output *85*
5.6.1 Different Methods of Analysis *85*
5.6.2 Likelihood and gee *85*
5.6.3 Interpreting Computer Output *86*
5.7 Model Checking *89*
5.8 Reporting the Results of Random Effects Analysis *89*
5.9 Reading about the Results of Random Effects Analysis *90*
5.10 Examples of Random Effects Models in the Medical Literature *90*
5.10.1 Cluster Trials *90*
5.10.2 Repeated Measures *91*
5.10.3 Comment *91*
5.10.4 Clustering in a Cohort Study *91*
5.10.5 Comment *91*
5.11 Frequently Asked Questions *91*
5.12 Exercises *92*

6 Poisson and Ordinal Regression *95*
6.1 Poisson Regression *95*
6.2 The Poisson Model *95*
6.3 Interpreting a Computer Output: Poisson Regression *96*
6.4 Model Checking for Poisson Regression *97*
6.5 Extensions to Poisson Regression *99*
6.6 Poisson Regression Used to Estimate Relative Risks from a 2 × 2 Table *99*
6.7 Poisson Regression in the Medical Literature *100*
6.8 Ordinal Regression *100*
6.9 Interpreting a Computer Output: Ordinal Regression *101*
6.10 Model Checking for Ordinal Regression *103*
6.11 Ordinal Regression in the Medical Literature *104*
6.12 Reporting the Results of Poisson or Ordinal Regression *104*
6.13 Reading about the Results of Poisson or Ordinal Regression *104*
6.14 Frequently Asked Question *105*
6.15 Exercises *105*

7 Meta-analysis *107*
7.1 Introduction *107*
7.2 Models for Meta-analysis *108*
7.3 Missing Values *111*
7.4 Displaying the Results of a Meta-analysis *111*
7.5 Interpreting a Computer Output *113*
7.6 Examples from the Medical Literature *114*
7.6.1 Example of a Meta-analysis of Clinical Trials *114*
7.6.2 Example of a Meta-analysis of Case-control Studies *115*
7.7 Reporting the Results of a Meta-analysis *115*
7.8 Reading about the Results of a Meta-analysis *116*
7.9 Frequently Asked Questions *116*
7.10 Exercise *118*

8 Time Series Regression *121*
8.1 Introduction *121*
8.2 The Model *122*
8.3 Estimation Using Correlated Residuals *122*
8.4 Interpreting a Computer Output: Time Series Regression *123*
8.5 Example of Time Series Regression in the Medical Literature *124*
8.6 Reporting the Results of Time Series Regression *125*
8.7 Reading about the Results of Time Series Regression *125*
8.8 Frequently Asked Questions *125*
8.9 Exercise *126*

Appendix 1 Exponentials and Logarithms *129*

Appendix 2 Maximum Likelihood and Significance Tests *133*
A2.1 Binomial Models and Likelihood *133*
A2.2 The Poisson Model *135*
A2.3 The Normal Model *135*
A2.4 Hypothesis Testing: the Likelihood Ratio Test *137*
A2.5 The Wald Test *138*
A2.6 The Score Test *138*
A2.7 Which Method to Choose? *139*
A2.8 Confidence Intervals *139*
A2.9 Deviance Residuals for Binary Data *140*
A2.10 Example: Derivation of the Deviances and Deviance Residuals Given in Table 3.3 *140*
A2.10.1 Grouped Data *140*
A2.10.2 Ungrouped Data *140*

Appendix 3 Bootstrapping and Variance Robust Standard Errors *143*
A3.1 The Bootstrap *143*
A3.2 Example of the Bootstrap *144*
A3.3 Interpreting a Computer Output: The Bootstrap *145*
A3.3.1 Two-sample T-test with Unequal Variances *145*
A3.4 The Bootstrap in the Medical Literature *145*
A3.5 Robust or Sandwich Estimate SEs *146*
A3.6 Interpreting a Computer Output: Robust SEs for Unequal Variances *147*
A3.7 Other Uses of Robust Regression *149*
A3.8 Reporting the Bootstrap and Robust SEs in the Literature *149*
A3.9 Frequently Asked Question *150*

Appendix 4 Bayesian Methods *151*
A4.1 Bayes' Theorem *151*
A4.2 Uses of Bayesian Methods *152*
A4.3 Computing in Bayes *153*
A4.4 Reading and Reporting Bayesian Methods in the Literature *154*
A4.5 Reading about the Results of Bayesian Methods in the Medical Literature *154*

Appendix 5 R codes *157*
A5.1 R Code for Chapter 2 *157*
A5.3 R Code for Chapter 3 *163*
A5.4 R Code for Chapter 4 *166*
A5.5 R Code for Chapter 5 *168*
A5.6 R Code for Chapter 6 *170*

A5.7 R Code for Chapter 7 *171*
A5.8 R Code for Chapter 8 *173*
A5.9 R Code for Appendix 1 *173*
A5.10 R Code for Appendix 2 *174*
A5.11 R Code for Appendix 3 *175*

Answers to Exercises *179*

Glossary *185*

Index *191*

Preface

In the 16 years since the second edition of *Statistics at Square Two* was published, there have been many developments in statistical methodology and in methods of presenting statistics. MJC is pleased that his colleague Richard Jacques, who has considerable experience in more advanced statistical methods and teaching medical statistics to non- statisticians, has joined him as a co-author. Most of the examples have been updated and two new chapters have been added on meta-analysis and on time series analysis. In addition, reference is made to the many checklists which have appeared since the last edition to enable better reporting of research.

This book is intended to build on the latest edition of *Statistics at Square One*.[1] It is hoped to be a *vade mecum* for investigators who have undergone a basic statistics course, but need more advanced methods. It is also intended for readers and users of the medical literature, but is intended to be rather more than a simple "bluffer's guide". It is hoped that it will encourage the user to seek professional help when necessary. Important sections in each chapter are tips on reading and reporting about a particular technique; the book emphasises correct interpretation of results in the literature. Much advanced statistical methodology is used rather uncritically in medical research, and the data and code to check whether the methods are valid are often not provided when the investigators write up their results. This text will help readers of statistics in medical research engage in constructive critical review of the literature.

Since most researchers do not want to become statisticians, detailed explanations of the methodology will be avoided. However, equations of the models are given, since they show concisely what each model is assuming. We hope the book will prove useful to students on postgraduate courses and for this reason there are a number of exercises with answers. For students on a more elementary course for health professionals we recommend Walters *et al.*[2]

The choice of topics reflects what we feel are commonly encountered in the medical literature, based on many years of statistical refereeing. The linking theme is regression models and we cover multiple regression, logistic regression, Cox regression, random effects (mixed models), ordinal regression, Poisson regression, time series regression and meta-analysis. The predominant philosophy is frequentist, since this reflects the literature and what is available in most packages. However, a discussion on the uses of Bayesian methods is given in an Appendix 4. The huge amount of work on causal modelling is briefly referenced, but is generally beyond the scope of this book.

Most of the concepts in statistical inference have been covered in *Statistics at Square One.*[1] In order to keep this book short, reference will be made to the earlier book for basic concepts. All the analyses described in the book have been conducted in the free software R and the code is given to make the methods accessible to reserachers without commercial statistical packages.

We are grateful to Tommy Nyberg of the Biostatistics Unit, Cambridge for feedback on his survival paper and to our colleague, Jeremy Dawson, who read and commented on the final draft. Any remaining errors are our own.

Michael J. Campbell
Richard M. Jacques
Sheffield, June 2022

References

1 Campbell MJ. *Statistics at Square One*, 12th edn. Hoboken, NJ: Wiley-Blackwell, 2021.
2 Walters SJ, Campbell MJ, Machin D. *Medical Statistics: A Textbook for the Health Sciences*, 5th edn. Chichester: John Wiley & Sons Ltd, 2020.

1

Models, Tests and Data

Summary

This chapter covers some of the basic concepts in statistical analysis, which are covered in greater depth in *Statistics at Square One*. It introduces the idea of a statistical model and then links it to statistical tests. The use of statistical models greatly expands the utility of statistical analysis. In particular, they allow the analyst to examine how a variety of variables may affect the result.

1.1 Types of Data

Data can be divided into two main types: quantitative and qualitative. *Quantitative data* tend to be either continuous variables that one can measure (such as height, weight or blood pressure) or discrete (such as numbers of children per family or numbers of attacks of asthma per child per month). Thus, count data are discrete and quantitative. Continuous variables are often described as having a Normal distribution, or being non-Normal. Having a Normal distribution means that if you plot a histogram of the data it would follow a particular "bell-shaped" curve. In practice, provided the data cluster about a single central point, and the distribution is symmetric about this point, it would be commonly considered close enough to Normal for most tests requiring Normality to be valid. Here one would expect the mean and median to be close. Non-Normal distributions tend to have asymmetric distributions (skewed) and the means and medians differ. Examples of non-Normally distributed variables include ages and salaries in a population. Sometimes the asymmetry is caused by outlying points that are in fact errors in the data and these need to be examined with care.

Note that it is a misnomer to talk of "non-parametric" data instead of non-Normally distributed data. Parameters belong to models, and what is meant by "non-parametric" data is data to which we cannot apply models, although as we shall see later, this is often a too limited view of statistical methods. An important feature of quantitative data is that you can deal with the numbers as having real meaning, so for example you can take averages of the data. This is in contrast to qualitative data, where the numbers are often convenient labels and have no quantitative value.

Qualitative data tend to be categories, thus people are male or female, European, American or Japanese, they have a disease or are in good health and can be described as

Statistics at Square Two: Understanding Modern Statistical Application in Medicine, Third Edition.
Michael J. Campbell and Richard M. Jacques.

nominal or *categorical*. If there are only two categories they are described as *binary* data. Sometimes the categories can be ordered, so for example a person can "get better", "stay the same" or "get worse". These are *ordinal* data. Often these will be scored, say, 1, 2, 3, but if you had two patients, one of whom got better and one of whom got worse, it makes no sense to say that on average they stayed the same (a statistician is someone with their head in the oven and their feet in the fridge, but on average they are comfortable!). The important feature about ordinal data is that they can be ordered, but there is no obvious weighting system. For example, it is unclear how to weight "healthy", "ill" or "dead" as outcomes. (Often, as we shall see later, either scoring by giving consecutive whole numbers to the ordered categories and treating the ordinal variable as a quantitative variable or dichotomising the variable and treating it as binary may work well.) Count data, such as numbers of children per family appear ordinal, but here the important feature is that arithmetic is possible (2.4 children per family is meaningful). This is sometimes described as having *ratio* properties. A family with four children has twice as many children as a family with two, but if we had an ordinal variable with four categories, say "strongly agree", "agree", "disagree" and "strongly disagree", and scored them 1–4, we cannot say that "strongly disagree", scored 4, is twice "agree", scored 2.

Qualitative data can also be formed by categorising continuous data. Thus, blood pressure is a continuous variable, but it can be split into "normotension" or "hypertension". This often makes it easier to summarise, for example 10% of the population have hypertension is easier to comprehend than a statement giving the mean and standard deviation of blood pressure in the population, although from the latter one could deduce the former (and more besides). Note that qualitative data is not necessarily associated with qualitative research. Qualitative research is of rising importance and complements quantitative research. The name derives because it does not quantify measures, but rather identifies themes, often using interviews and focus groups.

It is a parody to suggest that statisticians prefer not to dichotomise data and researchers always do it, but there is a grain of truth in it. Decisions are often binary: treat or not treat. It helps to have a "cut-off", for example treat with anti-hypertensive if diastolic blood pressure is >90 mmHg, although more experienced clinicians would take into account other factors related to the patient's condition and use the cut-off as a point when their likelihood of treating increases. However, statisticians point out the loss of information when data are dichotomised, and are also suspicious of arbitrary cut-offs, which may have been chosen to present a conclusion desired by a researcher. Although there may be good reasons for a cut-off, they are often opaque, for example deaths from Covid are defined as deaths occurring within 30 days of a positive Covid test. Why 30 days, and not 4 weeks (which would be easier to implement) or 3 months? Clearly ten years is too long. In this case it probably matters little which period of time is chosen but it shows how cut-offs are often required and the justification may be lost.

1.2 Confounding, Mediation and Effect Modification

Much medical research can be simplified as an investigation of an input–output relationship. The inputs, or explanatory variables, are thought to be related to the outcome or effect. We wish to investigate whether one or more of the input variables are plausibly causally related to the effect. The relationship is complicated by other factors that are thought to be related to both the cause and the effect; these are confounding factors. A simple example would be the relationship between stress and high blood pressure. Does stress cause high blood pressure? Here the causal variable is a measure of stress, which we assume can be quantified either as a binary or continuous variable, and the outcome is a blood pressure measurement. A confounding factor might be gender; men may be more prone to stress, but they may also be more prone to high blood pressure. If gender is a confounding factor, a study would need to take gender into account. A more precise definition of a confounder states that a confounder should "not be on the causal pathway". For example stress may cause people to drink more alcohol, and it is the increased alcohol consumption which causes high blood pressure. In this case alcohol consumption is not a confounder, and is often termed a *mediator*.

Another type of variable is an effect modifier. Again, it is easier to explain using an example. It is possible that older people are more likely than younger people to suffer high blood pressure when stressed. Age is not a confounder if older people are not more likely to be stressed than younger people. However, if we had two populations with different age distributions our estimate of the effect of stress on blood pressure would be different in the two populations if we didn't allow for age. Crudely, we wish to remove the effects of confounders, but study effect modifiers.

An important start in the analysis of data is to determine which variables are outputs and which variables are inputs, and of the latter which do we wish to investigate as causal, and which are confounders or effect modifiers. Of course, depending on the question, a variable might serve as any of these. In a survey of the effects of smoking on chronic bronchitis, smoking is a causal variable. In a clinical trial to examine the effects of cognitive behavioural therapy on smoking habit, smoking is an outcome. In the above study of stress and high blood pressure, smoking may also be a confounder.

A common error is to decide which of the variables are confounders by doing significance tests. One might see in a paper: "only variables that were significantly related to the output were included in the model." One issue with this is it makes it more difficult to repeat the research; a different researcher may get a different set of confounders. In later chapters we will discuss how this could go under the name of "stepwise" regression. We emphasise that significance tests are not a good method of choosing the variable to go in a model.

In summary, before any analysis is done, and preferably in the original protocol, the investigator should decide on the causal, outcome and confounder variables. An exploration of how variables relate in a model is given in Section 1.10.

1.3 Causal Inference

Causal inference is a new area of statistics that examines the relationship between a putative cause and an outcome. A useful and simple method of displaying a causal model is with a Direct Acyclic Graph (DAG).[1] They can be used to explain the definitions given in the previous section. There are two key features to DAGs: (1) they show direct relationships using lines and arrows and are usually read from left to right and (2) they don't allow feedback, that is, you can't get back to where you started following the arrows.

We start with a cause, which might be an exposure (E) or a treatment (T). This is related to an outcome (O) or disease (D) but often just denoted Y. Confounders (C) are variables related to both E and Y which may change the relationship between E and Y. In randomised trials, we can in theory remove the relationship between C and T by randomisation, so making causal inference is easier. For observational studies, we remove the link between C and T using models, but models are not reality and we may have omitted to measure key variables, so confounding and bias may still exist after modelling.

Figure 1.1 shows a simple example. We want to estimate the relationship between an exposure (E) and an outcome (O). C1 and C2 are confounders in that they may affect one another and they both affect E and O. Note that the direction of the arrows means that neither C1 nor C2 are affected by E or O. Thus, E could be stress as measured by the Perceived Stress Scale (PSS) and O could be high blood pressure. Then C1 could be age and C2 ethnicity. Although age and ethnicity are not causally related, in the UK ethnic minorities tend to be younger than the rest of the population. Older people and ethnic minorities may have more stress and have higher blood pressure for reasons other than stress. Thus, in a population that includes a wide range of ages and ethnicities we need to allow for these variable when considering whether stress causes high blood pressure.

An important condition for a variable to be a confounder is that it is not on the direct casual path. This is shown in Figure 1.2, where an intermediate variable (IM) is on the causal path between E and O. An example might be that stress causes people to drink alcohol and alcohol is the actual cause of high blood pressure. To control for alcohol, one might look at two models with different levels of drinking. One might fit a model with and without the intermediate factor, to see how the relationship between E and O changes.

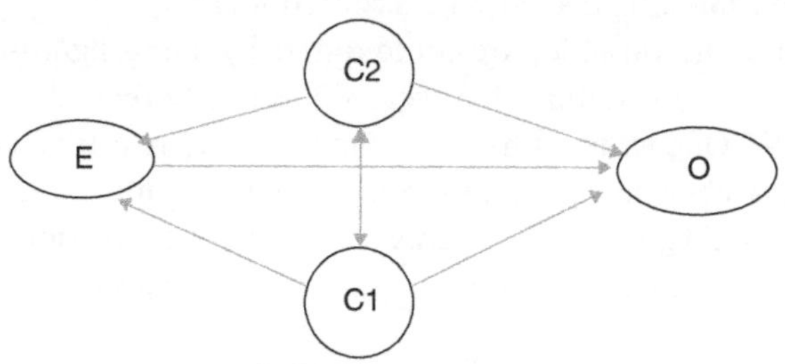

Figure 1.1 A DAG showing confounding.

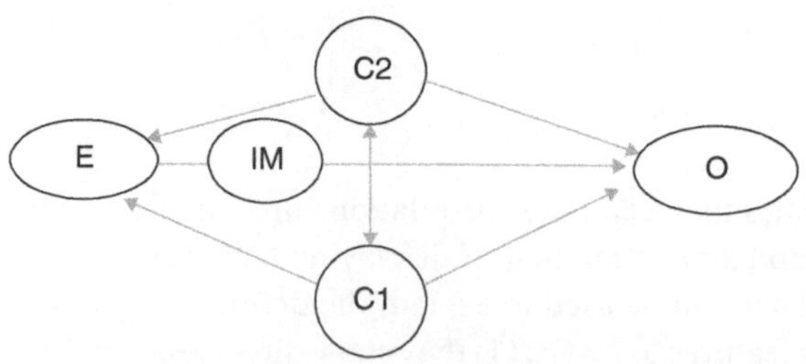

Figure 1.2 A DAG showing an intermediate variable (IM).

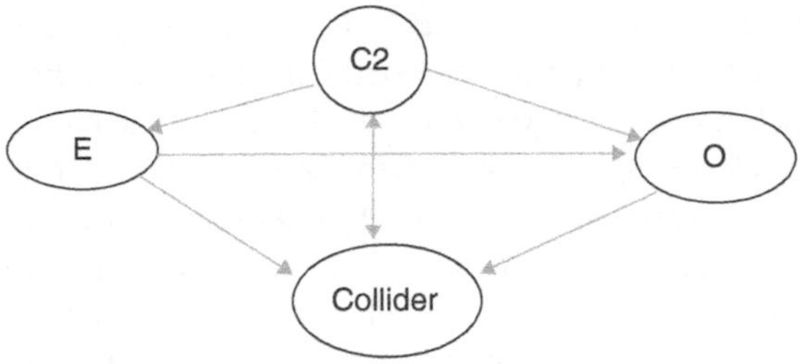

Figure 1.3 A DAG showing a collider.

One use of DAGs is to identify what is known as *Berkson's bias*. This is where the arrows are reversed going to one particular variable, and so they collide at this variable; this variable is called a *collider* (see Figure 1.3). This is the situation where having both O and E increases your chance of the collider. To extend the stress example, a hospital may run a cardiovascular clinic and so the investigators might choose cases of high blood pressure from the clinic and controls as people not in the clinic. However, stress may cause symptoms of cardiovascular disease and so stressed people are more likely to attend the clinic, which sets up a spurious association between stress and high blood pressure.

In general, allowing for confounders in models gives a better estimate of the strength of a causal relationship, whereas allowing for IMs and colliders does not and so it is important to identify which are which. DAGs are a qualitative way of expressing relationships, and one doesn't often see them in publications. They also have their limitations, such as in displaying effect modifiers.[2] Relationships can also depend on how a variable is coded, such as an absolute risk or a relative risk. Statistical models are useful for actually quantifying and clarifying these relationships.

1.4 Statistical Models

The relationship between inputs and outputs can be described by a mathematical model that relates the inputs, which we have described earlier with causal variables, confounders and effect modifiers (often called "independent variables" and denoted by X), with the output (often called "dependent variable" and denoted by Y). Thus, in the stress and blood pressure example above, we denote blood pressure by Y, and stress and gender are both X variables. Here the X does not distinguish between confounding and causality. We wish to know if stress is still a good predictor of blood pressure when we know an individual's gender. To do this we need to assume that gender and stress combine in some way to affect blood pressure. As discussed in *Statistics at Square One*, we describe the models at a *population* level. We take samples to get estimates of the population values. In general we will refer to population values using Greek letters and estimates using Roman letters.

The most commonly used models are known as "linear models". They assume that the X variables combine in a linear fashion to predict Y. Thus, if X_1 and X_2 are the two independent variables we assume that an equation of the form $\beta_0 + \beta_1X_1 + \beta_2X_2$ is the best predictor of Y where β_0, β_1 and β_2 are constants and are known as parameters of the model. The method often used for estimating the *parameters* is known as regression and so these are the *regression parameters*. The estimates are often referred to as the "regression coefficients". Slightly misleadingly, the X variables do not need to be independent of each other so another confounder in the stress/blood pressure relationship might be employment, and age and employment are related, so for example older people are more likely to be retired. This can be seen in Figure 1.1, where confounding variables may be linked. Another problem with the term "linear" is that it may include interactions, so the model may be of the form $\beta_0 + \beta_1X_1 + \beta_2X_2 + \beta_3X_1X_2$. An effect modifier, described in the previous section, may be modelled as an interaction between a possible cause X_1 and a possible confounder X_2.

Of course, no model can predict the Y variable perfectly and the model acknowledges this by incorporating an *error* term. These linear models are appropriate when the outcome variable is continuous. The wonderful aspect of these models is that they can be generalised so that the modelling procedure is similar for many different situations, such as when the outcome is non-Normal or discrete. Thus, different areas of statistics, such as t-tests and chi-squared tests are unified and dealt with in a similar manner using a method known as "generalised linear models".

When we have taken a sample, we can estimate the parameters of the model, and get a fit to the data. A simple description of the way that data relate to the model is given by Chatfield.[3]

$$\text{DATA} = \text{FIT} + \text{RESIDUAL}$$

The FIT is what is obtained from the model given the predictor variables. The RESIDUAL is the difference between the DATA and the FIT. For the linear model the residual is an estimate of the error term. For a generalised linear model this is not strictly the case, but the residual is useful for diagnosing poor fitting models, as we shall see later.

Models are used for two main purposes, *estimation* and *prediction*. For example we may wish to estimate the effect of stress on blood pressure, or predict what the lung function of an individual is given their age, height and gender.

Do not forget, however, that models are simply an approximation to reality. "All models are wrong, but some are useful."

The subsequent chapters describe different models where the dependent variable takes different forms: continuous, binary, a survival time, a count and ordinal and when the values are correlated such as when they are clustered or measurements are repeated on the same unit. A more advanced text covering similar material is that by Frank Harrell.[4] The rest of this chapter is a quick review of the basics covered in *Statistics at Square One*.

1.5 Results of Fitting Models

Models are fitted to data using a variety of methods. The oldest is the method of least squares, which finds values for the parameters that minimise the sum of the squared residuals. Another is *maximum likelihood*, which finds the values of the parameters that gives the highest *likelihood* of the data given the parameter estimates (see Appendix 2 for more details). For Normally distributed data the least squares method is also the maximum likelihood method. The output from a computer package will be an estimate of the parameter with an estimate of its variability (the standard error or SE). There will usually be a p-value and a confidence interval (CI) for the parameter. A further option is to use a *robust* standard error, or a *bootstrap standard error*, which are less dependent on the model assumptions and are described in Appendix 3. There will also be some measures as to whether the model is a good fit to the data.

1.6 Significance Tests

Significance tests such as the chi-squared test and the t-test, and the interpretation of p-values were described in *Statistics at Square One*. The usual format of statistical significance testing is to set up a *null hypothesis* and then collect data. Using the null hypothesis, we test if the observed data are consistent with the null hypothesis. As an example, consider a randomised clinical trial to compare a new diet with a standard diet to reduce weight in obese patients. The null hypothesis is that there is no difference between the two treatments in weight changes of the patients. The outcome is the difference in the mean weight after the two treatments. We can calculate the probability of getting the observed mean difference (or one more extreme), if the null hypothesis of no difference in the two diets is true. If this probability (the p-value) is sufficiently small we reject the null hypothesis and assume that the new diet differs from the standard. The usual method of doing this is to divide the mean difference in weight in the two diet groups by the estimated SE of the difference and compare this ratio to either a t-distribution (small sample) or a Normal distribution (large sample).

The test as described above is known as Student's t-test, but the form of the test, whereby an estimate is divided by its SE and compared to a Normal distribution, is known as a *Wald test* or a *z-test*.

There are, in fact, a large number of different types of statistical test. For Normally distributed data, they usually give the same p-values, but for other types of data they can give different results. In the medical literature there are three different tests that are commonly used, and it is important to be aware of the basis of their construction and their differences. These tests are known as the *Wald test*, the *score test* and the *likelihood ratio test*. For non-Normally distributed data, they can give different p-values, although usually the results converge as the data set increases in size. The basis for these three tests is described in Appendix 2.

In recent times there has been much controversy over significance tests.[5] They appear to answer a complex question with a simple answer, and as a consequence are often misused and misinterpreted. In particular, a non-significant p-value is supposed to indicate a lack of an effect, and a significant p-value to indicate an important effect. These misconceptions are discussed extensively in *Statistics at Square One*. The authors of this book believe they are still useful and so we will use them. It is one of our goals that this book will help reduce their misuse.

1.7 Confidence Intervals

One problem with statistical tests is that the p-value depends on the size of the data set. With a large enough data set, it would be almost always possible to prove that two treatments differed significantly, albeit by small amounts. It is important to present the results of an analysis with an estimate of the mean effect, and a measure of precision, such as a CI.[6] To understand a CI we need to consider the difference between a population and a sample. A population is a group to whom we make generalisations, such as patients with diabetes or middle-aged men. Populations have *parameters*, such as the mean HbA1c in people with diabetes or the mean blood pressure in middle-aged men. Models are used to model populations and so the parameters in a model are population parameters. We take samples to get *estimates* for model parameters. We cannot expect the estimate of a model parameter to be exactly equal to the true model parameter, but as the sample gets larger we would expect the estimate to get closer to the true value, and a CI about the estimate helps to quantify this. A 95% CI for a population mean implies that if we took 100 samples of a fixed size, and calculated the mean and 95% CI for each, then we would expect 95 of the intervals to include the true population parameter. The way they are commonly understood from a single sample is that there is a 95% chance that the population parameter is in the 95% CI. Another way of interpreting a CI is to say it is a set of values of the null hypothesis, from which the observed data would not be statistically significant. This points out that just as there are three commonly used methods to find p-values, there are also a number of different methods to find CIs, and the method should be stated.[6]

In the diet trial example given above, the CI will measure how precisely we can estimate the effect of the new diet. If in fact the new diet were no different from the old, we would expect the CI for the effect measure to contain 0.

Cynics sometimes say that a CI is often used as a proxy for a significance test, that is, the writer simply reports whether the CI includes the null hypothesis. However, using CIs emphasises *estimation* rather than *tests* and we believe this is the important goal of analysis, that is, it is better to say being vaccinated reduces your risk of catching Covid by a factor of 95% (95% CI 90.3 to 97.6) than to simply say vaccination protects you from Covid ($P < 0.001$).[7]

CIs are also useful in *non-inferiority* studies, where one might want to show that two treatments are effectively equivalent, but perhaps one has fewer side effects than the other. Here one has to specify a non-inferiority margin, and conclude non-inferiority if the CI does not include the margin but does include a difference of zero. The concepts of null and alternative hypotheses are reversed and so require careful thought. Further discussion is given, for example, by Hahn.[8]

1.8 Statistical Tests Using Models

A t-test compares the mean values of a continuous variable in two groups. This can be written as a linear model. In the example of the trial of two diets given above, weight after treatment was the continuous variable. Here the primary predictor variable X is Diet, which is a binary variable taking the value (say) 0 for the standard diet and 1 for the new diet. The outcome variable is weight. There are no confounding variables (in theory because this is a randomised trial). The fitted model is Weight $= b_0 + b_1 \times$ Diet + Residual. The FIT part of the model is $b_0 + b_1 \times$ Diet and is what we would predict someone's weight to be given our estimate of the effect of the diet. We assume that the residuals have an approximate Normal distribution. The null hypothesis is that the coefficient associated with diet b_1 is from a population with mean 0. Thus, we assume that β_1, the population parameter, is 0 and, rather than using a simple test, we can use a model. The results from a t-test and linear regression are compared in Appendix 3.

Models enable us to make our assumptions explicit. A nice feature about models, as opposed to tests, is that they are easily extended. Thus, weight at baseline may (by chance) differ in the two groups, and will be related to weight after treatment, so it could be included as a confounder variable. Similarly, smoking may be an effect modifier and so that could be included in the model as well.

This method is further described in Chapter 2 as multiple regression. The treatment of the chi-squared test as a model is described in Chapter 3 under logistic regression.

1.9 Many Variables

It may seem merely semantic but it is useful to distinguish between *multivariate* and *multivariable* analysis.[9] A multivariable model can be thought of as a model in which multiple variables are found on the right side of the model equation. This type of statistical model can be used to attempt to assess the relationship between a number of variables; one can assess independent relationships while adjusting for potential confounders. There is only one outcome variable. For models such as linear regression, the generalisation with many predictors is known as *multiple linear regression*.

Multivariate, by contrast, refers to the modelling of data that are often derived from longitudinal studies, wherein an outcome is measured for the same individual at multiple time points (repeated measures), or the modelling of nested/clustered data, wherein there are multiple individuals in each cluster. Techniques for multivariate analysis include *factor analysis, cluster methods* and *discriminant analysis*. In this book, we are more interested in analyses where there is only one outcome measure and a variety of possible predictor variables which can be combined into a prediction, and so we do not consider multivariate methods. Thus, it is a misnomer to call techniques such as multivariable regression as *multivariate* since there is only one outcome variable and so it is better to refer to multiple linear regression (Chapter 2) and similarly with multiple logistic regression (Chapter 3).

Using a multivariable model means we can estimate the relationship between exposure (E) and outcome (O) in Figure 1.1 *controlling* for the confounders C_1 and C_2. For example, in an observational study, a confounder may be age, and the age distribution for those exposed may be different from that of those not exposed. We can use a multivariable model to estimate the relationship between E and O *allowing for* age. Similarly, we can explore how different variables interact when predicting the outcome variable. In a clinical trial, we can explore whether the treatment effect varies by (pre-specified) subgroups. We can use models for prediction, for example predict lung function given a person's personal characteristics. The great advantage of a model is that we can predict what a particular person's expected lung function should be, given say their age, height, gender and smoking habit *even though* a person with these precise characteristics is not in the data set.

A reader should always question why covariates are included in a regression.[10] A common error is to only include covariates which are statistically significantly related to the exposure in the model. In clinical trials, the reason is that randomisation, if done correctly, will have rendered the relationship between a treatment and a covariate null, and any observed difference will, by definition, be due to chance. A more fundamental reason is that such a test does not tell us whether the covariate should be included; non-significant covariates can be important effect modifiers and covariates may act by interaction with other covariates which singular testing would not reveal. It also makes the study more difficult to repeat; should a new investigator choose covariates which a previous investigator found by individual testing, even if they are not significant in the second study? The usual advice is to pre-specify the covariates to be used in a study but this is sometimes to assign divine knowledge to the investigator, who will want to discover relationships not previously anticipated. It can help to decide on whether the study is *explanatory* or *confirmatory*, as explained in Section 1.10.

1.10 Model Fitting and Analysis: Exploratory and Confirmatory Analyses

There are two aspects to data analysis: confirmatory and exploratory analyses. In a *confirmatory analysis* we are testing a pre-specified hypothesis and it follows naturally to conduct significance tests. Testing for a treatment effect in a clinical trial is a good example of a confirmatory analysis. In an *exploratory analysis* we are looking to see what the data are telling us. An example would be looking for risk factors in a cohort study. A technique such as *stepwise* regression, which tries to find the best fitting model out of a set of covariates, is an example of an explanatory technique. The findings should be regarded as tentative to be confirmed in a subsequent study, and p-values are largely decorative.

Often one can do both types of analysis in the same study. For example, when analysing a clinical trial, a large number of possible outcomes may have been measured. Those specified in the protocol as primary outcomes are subjected to a confirmatory analysis, but there is often a large amount of information, say concerning side effects, which could also be analysed. These should be reported, but with a warning that they emerged from the analysis and not from a pre-specified hypothesis. It seems illogical to ignore information in a study, but also the lure of an apparent unexpected significant result can be very difficult to resist (but should be).

It may also be useful to distinguish *audit*, which is largely descriptive, intending to provide information about one particular time and place, and *research*, which tries to be generalisable to other times and places.

1.11 Computer-intensive Methods

Much of the theory described in the rest of this book requires some prescription of a distribution for the data, such as the Normal distribution. There are now methods available which use models but are less dependent on the actual distribution of the data. They are commonly available in computer packages and are easy to use. A description of one such method, the bootstrap, is given in Appendix 3.1. For *prediction*, there are now many methods which include *machine learning* or *artificial intelligence*, for example to predict Covid-19 progression.[11] They eschew a fixed model, and instead learn from many combinations of the data to find which combinations give the best predictions. An advantage of these methods is that real life does not behave like a model and so they may be better at predicting events than trying to find a model to do so. The problem with these methods is that because they are "black-box" they don't really explain how their inputs relate to each other, and their predictions are often not associated with measures of uncertainty. In future, they may replace models, but not as yet since their utility is still being explored.

1.12 Missing Values

Missing values are the bane of a statistical analyst's life and are usually not discussed in elementary textbooks. In any survey, for example, some people will not respond; at worst we need to know how many are missing and at best we would like some data on them, say their age and gender. Then we can make some elementary checks to see if the subjects who did respond are typical. (One usually finds that the worst responders are young and male). One then has to decide whether anything needs to be done. For longitudinal data, it is important to distinguish values missing in the main outcome variables and values missing in covariates. For the outcome variables, missing values are often characterised into one of three groups: (1) missing completely at random (MCAR); (2) missing at random (MAR) and (3) not missing at random (NMAR) or non-ignorable (NI).[12] The crucial difference between (1) and (2) is that for (2) the reason for a value being missing can depend on previously recorded input and outcome variables, but must not depend on the value that is missing beyond what can be explained by other variables in the model. Thus a blood pressure value would be NMAR (NI) if it were missing every time the blood pressure exceeded 180 mmHg (which we cannot measure but can say that it made the patient too ill to turn up). However, if it were missing because the previous value exceeded 180 mmHg and the patient was then taken out of the study then it may be MAR. The important point to be made is that the reason for missing in MAR is independent of the actual value of the observation *conditional* on previous observations.

In longitudinal clinical trials it used to be traditional to ignore subjects if the values were missing. However, this can lead to biased and inefficient treatment estimates. The usual method of dealing with missing values is called *last observation carried forward* (LOCF), which does exactly what it says. However, this can also lead to bias and a number of other techniques have been developed including *imputation*, where the missing value is guessed from other values. *Multiple imputation* gives a distribution of possible values and enables uncertainty about the missing values to be incorporated in the analysis. The use of random effects models is also a way of analysing all the data measured for some longitudinal designs (see Chapter 5). Care, thought and sensitivity analyses are needed with missing data. For further details see, for example, Little and Rubin.[12]

1.13 Bayesian Methods

The model-based approach to statistics leads one to statements such as: "given model M, the probability of obtaining data D is P." This is known as the *frequentist* approach. This assumes that population parameters are fixed. However, many investigators would like to make statements about the probability of model M being true, in the form "given the data D, what is the probability that model M is the correct one?" Thus, one would like to know, for example, what is the probability of a diet working. A statement of this form would be particularly helpful for people who have to make decisions about individual patients. This leads to a way of thinking known as "Bayesian", which allows population parameters to vary. It has particular uses in health economics and health decision making where we would like to know the probability of a drug being cost effective.[13] Bayesian thinking is often facilitated by the use of DAGs.

This book is largely based on the frequentist approach. Most computer packages are also based on this approach, although most now enable Bayesian analysis as well. Further discussion on Bayesian methods is given in Chapter 5 and Appendix 4.

1.14 Causal Modelling

The models described earlier could be described as causal models. However, there is a specific area of *causal modelling* which is increasingly becoming more prevalent in biomedicine. It is beyond the scope of this book and here we just mention some areas that we have used in our own research, so that the reader will recognise them when reading the medical literature.

The models described in this book have the dependent variable on the left of the equation and the independent variables on the right. In econometrics the independent variables are termed *exogenous* and the dependent variables *endogenous* (probably better terms than the ones used here) and econometricians have long dealt with the observational data where the endogenous variables can be on the right-hand side as well. For example, consider a series of cross-sectional studies of children where we are interested in obesity.[14] We may be interested in factors influencing the obesity of children at age seven conditional of the obesity of the children when they were younger. The interest is obesity at age seven, but obesity at younger ages are endogenous variables to be included in the model. Each endogenous variable will have its own set of predictor (exogenous) variables, which gives a series of simultaneous equations. This is known as a *structural equation model*. These models often look at concepts which cannot be observed directly, or are measured with error. These are known as *latent variables*. For example Grey *et al.*[14] considered "family lifestyle" as a latent variable. They concluded that family lifestyle has a significant influence on all outcomes in their study, including diet, exercise and parental weight status. Family lifestyle accounted for 11.3% of the variation in child weight by the age of seven.

A useful philosophical idea for thinking about causality is that of the *counterfactual*, that is, consider two parallel universes: in one universe a person gets a treatment and in the other they get a control. The difference in outcomes for the *same* person is the effect of treatment. The closest we can get to this is a cross-over trial, where we randomise the order of treatment to a single person, but this requires that after the first treatment the person can return to a pre-treatment state before receiving the second. The next closest is a parallel randomised trial. Counterfactuals are used in treatment switching trials, comparing two treatments and where the length of survival is the outcome.[15] Data gathered earlier in the trial might indicate that one treatment is superior to the another and so all patients still in the trial are switched to the superior treatment. However, to estimate the cost-benefit of treatment we would wish to know how long people would have survived *if* they had stayed on the original treatment and so need to estimate the counterfactual using some form of predictive model based on patient characteristics.

A common problem in observational data is to evaluate a treatment where randomisation is not possible. Consider a study of the effect of breastfeeding of babies on the obesity of the child seven years later.[14] The issue is that there are confounding factors that determine whether a mother breastfeeds which may also determine whether the child is subsequently obese, such as income or education. This is usually tackled using linear or logistic regression which are discussed in Chapters 2 and 3. However, an alternative method is to use *propensity scores*.[16] Here models use the characteristics of a mother to predict the probability that she will breastfeed. Mothers who breastfeed are then matched with those who don't and a measure of obesity such as the body mass index of the children at seven are compared. There are various methods of matching, including pair matching, stratification of the propensity score or the use of the score as a covariate in a regression model. Propensity score methods rely on the assumption that we have measured *all* the covariates that determine breastfeeding to give unbiased results.[17] Some empirical studies, comparing estimates obtained from observational data using propensity scores and those from conventional trials, have shown that trials show more modest effects than estimates using propensity scores.[17] Traditional epidemiologists are very cautious about the term "causal" and will invoke criteria such as those of Bradford-Hill to bolster their claims. These criteria include the strength of the relationship, the plausibility of it, a dose response and the exposure must come before the outcome (temporality). For a discussion of how these criteria work in modern molecular biology, see the article by Fedak *et al.*[18] In trials where randomisation occurs, there are fewer inhibitions in making conclusions but it is perhaps unfortunate that some users of propensity score methods, which are, after all, based on observational data, take on the confident tone of trialist with regard to causality.

The whole issue of causal modelling can become rather "black-box" where insight as to how inferences are obtained can rest on many unacknowledged assumptions. For further reading see, for example, Imbens and Rubin.[19]

1.15 Reporting Statistical Results in the Medical Literature

The reporting of statistical results in the medical literature often leaves something to be desired. Here we will briefly give some tips that can be generally applied. In subsequent chapters we will consider specialised analyses.

Lang and Secic[20] give an excellent description of a variety of methods for reporting statistics in the medical literature. Checklists for reading and reporting statistical analyses are also given in Mansournia *et al.*[21] A huge variety of checklists for reporting results from different types of study are given on the Equator website.[22] These include the CONSORT statement for clinical trials[23] and the STROBE statement for observational studies.[24]

- Always describe how the subjects were recruited and how many were entered into the study and how many dropped out. For clinical trials one should say how many were screened for entry and describe the drop-outs by treatment group.
- Describe the model used and assumptions underlying the model and how these were verified. Always give an estimate of the main effect, with a measure of precision, such as a 95% CI as well as the p-value. It is important to give the right estimate. Thus, in a clinical trial, while it is of interest to have the mean of the outcome, by treatment group, the main measure of the effect is the difference in means and a CI for the difference. This can often not be derived from the CIs of the means for each treatment.
- It is often sensible to apply several models for the same data to show how including variables changes the model estimates. In the stress example, give the coefficients for separate models allowing sequentially for, for example, gender and alcohol consumption, and by age.
- Describe how the p-values were obtained (Wald, likelihood ratio or score) or the actual tests and similarly with CIs.
- It is sometimes useful to describe the data using binary data (e.g. percentage of people with hypertension), but analyse the continuous measurement (e.g. blood pressure).
- Describe which computer package was used. This will often explain why a particular test was used. Results from "home-grown" programs may need further verification. It is very helpful to make the code and data available for future analysts.

1.16 Reading Statistics in the Medical Literature

- From what population are the data drawn? Are the results generalisable?
- Can you tell how much of the original data collected appeared in the report and was it a high proportion? Did many people refuse to cooperate? Were missing values investigated using imputation or sensitivity analyses?
- Is the analysis confirmatory or exploratory? Is it research or audit?
- Have the correct statistical models been used?
- Do not be satisfied with statements such as, "a significant effect was found". Ask what is the size of the effect and will it make a difference to patients (often described as a "clinically significant effect")?
- Verify that the assumptions of the model are met. For example, if a linear model is used, what evidence is there for linearity. If paired data are used, is pairing reflected in the analysis?

- Are the results critically dependent on the assumptions about the models? Often the results are quite "robust" to the actual model, but this needs to be considered. For example if the data set is large the assumption of Normality for residuals is less critical.
- How were the confounders chosen? As stated earlier it is a classic mistake to use individual significance tests to see whether a potential confounder differs between treatment and control (in a trial) or between exposed and not exposed (in an observational study). The problem is that the significance test does not tell us whether a variable should be included in a model. Ideally, variables used in a model should be specified in advance. However, this may not be possible, and the analysis should be described as *exploratory*.
- Were different models shown with and without possible confounders to describe the effects of confounding and effect modification?

References

1 Greenland S, Pearl J, Robins J. Causal diagrams for epidemiologic research. *Epidemiology* 1999; **10**: 37–48.

2 Weinberg CR. Can DAGs clarify effect modification? *Epidemiology* 2007; **18**(5): 569–72. doi: 10.1097/EDE.0b013e318126c11d

3 Chatfield C. *Problem Solving: A Statistician's Guide*. London: Chapman and Hall, 1995.

4 Harrell FE. *Regression Modeling Strategies with Applications to Linear Models, Logistic and Ordinal Regression and Survival Analysis*. New York: Wiley, Springer Series is Statistics, 2015.

5 Wasserstein RL, Lazar NA. The ASA's statement on p-values: context, process and purpose. *Am Stat* 2016; **70**: 129–33.

6 Altman D, Machin D, Bryant T, Gardner M, eds. *Statistics with Confidence: Confidence Intervals and Statistical Guidelines*. Chichester: John Wiley & Sons, 2013.

7 Polack FP, Thomas SJ, Kitchin N, *et al*. Safety and efficacy of the BNT162b2 mRNA Covid-19 vaccine. *N Engl J Med* 2020; **383**: 2603–15.

8 Hahn S. Understanding non-inferiority trials. *Korean J Pediatr* 2012; **55**(11): 403–7. doi: 10.3345/kjp.2012.55.11.403

9 Hidalgo B, Goodman M. Multivariate or multivariable regression? *Am J Public Health* 2013; **103**(1): 39–40.

10 Nojima M, Tokunaga M, Nagamura F. Quantitative investigation of inappropriate regression model construction and the importance of medical statistics experts in observational medical research: a cross-sectional study. *BMJ Open* 2018; **8**: e021129. doi: 10.1136/bmjopen-2017-021129

11 Painuli D, Mishra D, Bhardwaj S, Aggarwal M. Forecast and prediction of COVID-19 using machine learning. *Data Science for COVID-19* 2021; 381–97. doi: 10.1016/B978-0-12-824536-1.00027-7

12 Little RJA, Rubin DB. *Statistical Analysis with Missing Data*. Chichester: John Wiley, 2019.

13 Baio G. *Bayesian Methods in Health Economics*. Boca Raton, FL: CRC Press, 2013.

14 Gray LA, Alava MH, Kelly MP, Campbell MJ. Family lifestyle dynamics and childhood obesity: evidence from the millennium cohort study. *BMC Public Health* 2018; **18**(1): 500.

15 Latimer NR, Abrams KR, Lambert PC, *et al.* Adjusting for treatment switching in randomised controlled trials–a simulation study and a simplified two-stage method. *Stat Methods Med Res* 2017; **26**(2): 724–51.

16 Gibson LA, Hernández Alava M, Kelly MP, Campbell MJ. The effects of breastfeeding on childhood BMI: a propensity score matching approach. *J Public Health* 2017; **39**(4): e152–60.

17 Campbell MJ. What is propensity score modelling? *Emerg Med J* 2017; **34**: 129–31. doi: 10.1136/emermed-2016-206542

18 Fedak KM, Bernal A, Capshaw ZA, Gross S. Applying the Bradford Hill criteria in the 21st century: how data integration has changed causal inference in molecular epidemiology. *Emerg Themes Epidemiol* 2015; **12**: 14. doi: 10.1186/s12982-015-0037-4

19 Imbens GW, Rubin DB. *Causal Inference for Statistics, Social, and Biomedical Sciences.* Cambridge: Cambridge University Press, 2015.

20 Lang TA, Secic M. *How to Report Statistics in Medicine: Annotated Guidelines for Authors, Editors and Reviewers.* Philadelphia, PA: American College of Physicians, 2006.

21 Mansournia MA, Collins GS, Nielsen RO, *et al.* A checklist for statistical assessment of medical papers (the CHAMP statement): explanation and elaboration. *Br J Sports Med* 2021; **55**: 1009–17. doi: 10.1136/bjsports-2020-103652

22 The EQUATOR Network. Enhancing the QUAlity and Transparency Of Health Research (equator-network.org)

23 CONSORT Consort – Welcome to the CONSORT Website (www.consort-statement.org)

24 STROBE Checklists – STROBE (www.strobe-statement.org)

2

Multiple Linear Regression

Summary

When we wish to model a continuous outcome variable, then an appropriate analysis is often *multiple linear regression*. For simple linear regression we have one continuous input variable.[1] In multiple regression we generalise the method to more than one input variable and we allow them to be continuous or nominal. We will discuss the use of *dummy* or *indicator variables* to model categories and investigate the sensitivity of models to individual data points using concepts such as *leverage* and *influence*. Multiple regression is a generalisation of the *analysis of variance* and *analysis of covariance*. The modelling techniques used here will be useful for the subsequent chapters.

2.1 The Model

In multiple regression the basic model is the following:

$$y_i = \beta_0 + \beta_1 X_{i1} + \beta_2 X_{i2} + \ldots + \beta_p X_{ip} + \varepsilon_i \tag{2.1}$$

We assume that the error term ε_i is Normally distributed, with mean 0 and standard deviation (s.d.) σ.

In terms of the model structure described in Chapter 1, the link is a linear one and the error term is Normal.

Here, y_i is the output for unit or subject i and there are p input variables $X_{i1}, X_{i2}, \ldots, X_{ip}$. Often y_i is termed the *dependent* variable and the input variables $X_{i1}, X_{i2}, \ldots, X_{ip}$ are termed the *independent variables*. The latter can be continuous or nominal. However, the term "independent" is a misnomer since the Xs need not be independent of each other. Sometimes they are called the *explanatory* or *predictor* variables. Each of the input variables is associated with a *regression coefficient* $\beta_1, \beta_2, \ldots, \beta_p$. There is also an additive constant term β_0. These are the *model parameters*.

Statistics at Square Two: Understanding Modern Statistical Application in Medicine, Third Edition.
Michael J. Campbell and Richard M. Jacques.

We can write the first section on the right hand side of Equation 2.1 as:

$$LP_i = \beta_0 + \beta_1 X_{i1} + \beta_2 X_{i2} + \ldots + \beta_p X_{ip}$$

where LP_i is known as the *linear predictor* and is the value of y_i predicted by the input variables. The difference $y_i - LP_i = \varepsilon_i$ is the *error* term.

The models are fitted by choosing estimates $b_0, b_1, \ldots, b_p$ which minimise the sum of squares (SS) of the predicted error. These estimates are termed *ordinary least squares* estimates. Using these estimates we can calculate the fitted values y_i^{fit} and the observed residuals $e_i = y_i - y_i^{fit}$ as discussed in Chapter 1. Here it is clear that the residuals estimate the error term. Further details are given in, for example, Draper and Smith.[2]

2.2 Uses of Multiple Regression

Multiple regression is one of the most useful tools in a statistician's armoury.

1) To estimate the relationship between an input (independent) variable and a continuous output (dependent) variable adjusting for the effects of potential confounding variables. For example, to investigate the effect of diet on weight allowing for smoking habits. Here the dependent variable is the outcome from a clinical trial. The independent variables could be the two treatment groups (as a 0/1 binary variable), smoking (as a continuous variable in numbers of packs per week) and baseline weight. The multiple regression model allows one to compare the outcome between groups, having adjusted for differences in baseline weight and smoking habit. This is also known as *analysis of covariance*.
2) To analyse the simultaneous effects of a number of categorical variables on a continuous output variable. An alternative technique is the *analysis of variance* but the same results can be achieved using multiple regression.
3) To predict a value of a continuous outcome for given inputs. For example, an investigator might wish to predict the forced expiratory volume (FEV_1) of a subject given age and height, so as to be able to calculate the observed FEV_1 as a percentage of predicted, and to decide if the observed FEV_1 is below, say, 80% of the predicted one.

2.3 Two Independent Variables

We will start off by considering two independent variables, which can be either continuous or binary. There are three possibilities: both variables continuous, both binary (0/1), or one continuous and one binary. We will anchor the examples in some real data.

Example

Consider the data given on the pulmonary anatomical deadspace and height in 15 children given in Campbell.[1] Suppose that of the 15 children, 8 had asthma and 4 bronchitis. The data are given in Table 2.1.

Table 2.1 Lung function data on 15 children.

Child	Deadspace	Height	Asthma	Age	Bronchitis
Number	(ml)	(cm)	(0 no, 1 yes)	(years)	(0 no, 1 yes)
1	44	110	1	5	0
2	31	116	0	5	1
3	43	124	1	6	0
4	45	129	1	7	0
5	56	131	1	7	0
6	79	138	0	6	0
7	57	142	1	6	0
8	56	150	1	8	0
9	58	153	1	8	0
10	92	155	0	9	1
11	78	156	0	7	1
12	64	159	1	8	0
13	88	164	0	10	1
14	112	168	0	11	0
15	101	174	0	14	0

Data from [1].

2.3.1 One Continuous and One Binary Independent Variable

In Campbell[1] the question posed was whether there is a relationship between deadspace and height. Here we might ask, is there a different relationship between deadspace and height for children with and without asthma?

Suppose the two independent variables are height and asthma status. There are a number of possible models:

1) *The slope and the intercept are the same for the two groups even though the means are different.* The model is:

$$\text{Deadspace} = \beta_0 + \beta_{\text{Height}} \times \text{Height} \tag{2.2}$$

This is illustrated in Figure 2.1. This is the simple linear regression model described in Campbell (Chapter 11).[1]

2) *The slopes are the same, but the intercepts are different.*
The model is:

$$\text{Deadspace} = \beta_0 + \beta_{\text{Height}} \times \text{Height} + \beta_{\text{Asthma}} \times \text{Asthma} \tag{2.3}$$

This is illustrated in Figure 2.2.

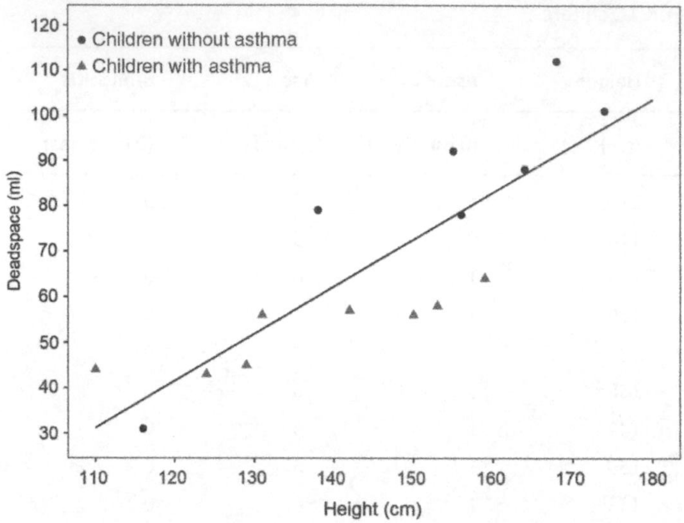

Figure 2.1 Deadspace versus height, ignoring asthma status. *Source:* [1] / John Wiley & Sons.

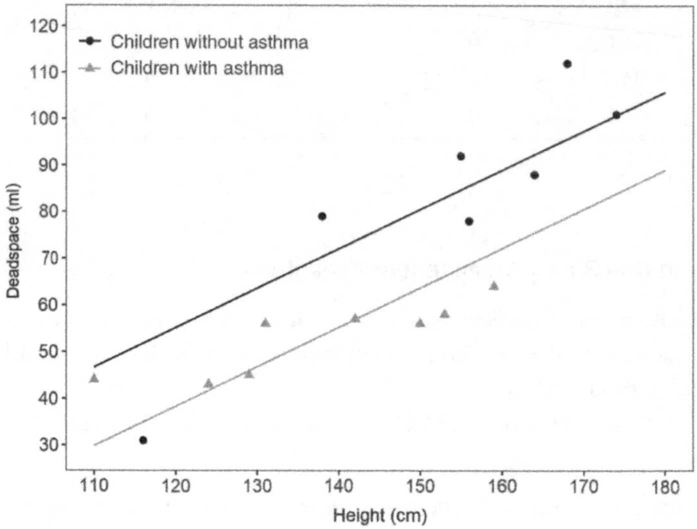

Figure 2.2 Parallel slopes for children with and without asthma.

It can be seen from model 2.3 that the interpretation of the coefficient β_{Asthma} is the difference in the intercepts of the two parallel lines which have slope β_{Height}. It is the difference in deadspace between children with and without asthma for any value of height, or in other words, it is the difference *allowing for* height. Thus if we thought that the only reason that children with and without asthma in our sample differed in the deadspace was because of a difference in height, then this is the sort of model we would fit. This type of model is termed an *analysis of covariance*. It is very common in the medical literature. An important assumption is that the slope is the same for the two groups.

We shall see later that, although they have the same symbol, we will get different estimates of β_{Height} when we fit Equations 2.2 and 2.3.

3) *The slopes and the intercepts are different in each group.*
   To model this we form a third variable x_3 = Height × Asthma. Thus x_3 is the same as height when the subject has asthma and is 0 otherwise. The variable x_3 measures the *interaction* between asthma status and height. It measures by how much the slope between deadspace and height is affected by having asthma.
   The model is:

$$\text{Deadspace} = \beta_0 + \beta_{\text{Height}} \times \text{Height} + \beta_{\text{Asthma}} \times \text{Asthma} + \beta_3 \times \text{Height} \times \text{Asthma} \quad (2.4)$$

This is illustrated in Figure 2.3, in which we have separate slopes for children with and without asthma.

The two lines are:

Children without asthma:

$$\text{Group} = 0: \text{Deadspace} = \beta_0 + \beta_{\text{Height}} \times \text{Height}$$

Children with asthma:

$$\text{Group} = 1: \text{Deadspace} = (\beta_0 + \beta_{\text{Asthma}}) + (\beta_{\text{Height}} + \beta_3) \times \text{Height}$$

In this model the interpretation of β_{Height} has changed from model 2.3. It is now the slope of the expected line for children without asthma. The slope of the line for children with asthma is $\beta_{\text{Height}} + \beta_3$. We then get the difference in slopes between children with and without asthma given by β_3.

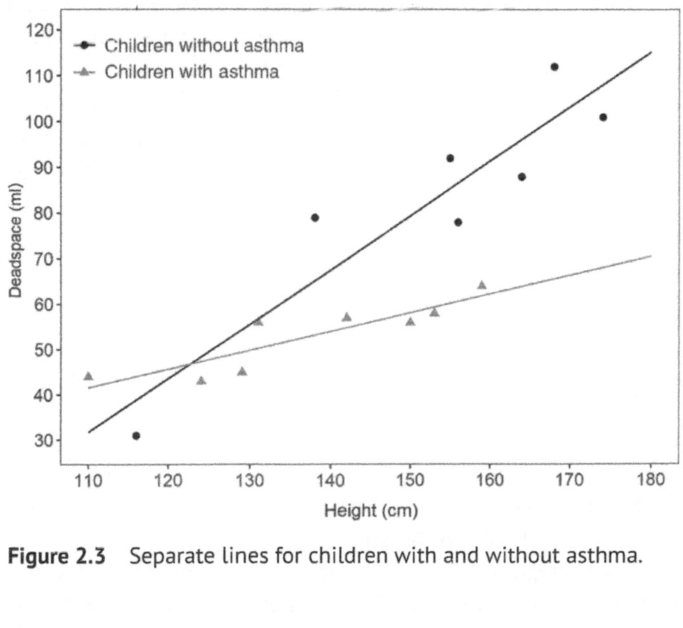

Figure 2.3 Separate lines for children with and without asthma.

2.3.2 Two Continuous Independent Variables

As an example of a situation where both independent variables are continuous, consider the data given in Table 2.1, but suppose we were interested in whether height and age together were important in the prediction of deadspace. The equation is:

$$\text{Deadspace} = \beta_0 + \beta_{\text{Height}} \times \text{Height} + \beta_{\text{Age}} \times \text{Age} \quad (2.5)$$

The interpretation of this model is trickier than the earlier one and the graphical visualisation is more difficult. We have to imagine that we have a whole variety of subjects all of the same age, but of different heights. Then we expect the deadspace to go up by β_{Height} (ml) for each centimetre in height, irrespective of the age of the subjects. We also have to imagine a group of subjects, all of the same height, but different ages. Then we expect the deadspace to go up by β_{Age} (ml) for each year of age, irrespective of the heights of the subjects. The nice feature of this model is that we can estimate these coefficients reasonably even if none of the subjects has exactly the same age or height.

If age and height were independent of each other then we can reasonably expect the β_{Height} in Equation 2.2 to be close to the β_{Height} in Equation 2.5, but clearly in this case age and height are not independent.

This model is commonly used in prediction as described in Section 2.2.

Some authors and some statistical packages compute regressions on what are called standardised variables, which are defined as:

$$\textit{Standardised}(x) = \frac{x - \textit{mean}(x)}{\textit{Standard deviation}(x)}$$

These are computed on both dependent and independent variables. Sometimes these are referred to as *z-scores*. The advantage of these is that one can compare coefficients directly, so in theory the larger the regression coefficient for a standardised covariate the larger its importance. Since they are merely scaling factors they do not change the t-statistic or p-value associated with the covariate. Confusingly they are also used with binary covariates, which destroys the simple interpretation of the coefficient associated with a binary covariate. (Although the s.d. of a proportion p if $0.2 < p < 0.8$ is approximately 0.5 so one would expect the coefficient for a standardised binary covariate to be about half that for non-standardised one.) Also, confusingly some statistical packages (e.g. SPSS) label the non-standardised coefficients B and the standardised ones β, a symbol usually reserved for the population value.

2.3.3 Categorical Independent Variables

In Table 2.1 the way that asthma status was coded is known as a *dummy* or *indicator* variable. The status has two levels, children with and without asthma, and just one dummy variable, the coefficient of which measures the difference in the *y* variable between children with and without asthma. For inference it does not matter if we code 1 for children with asthma and 0 for children without asthma or vice versa. The only effect is to change the sign of the coefficient; the p-value will remain the same.

However, Table 2.1 describes two categories of disease: asthma and bronchitis. If a subject has neither they will be taken as normal even though there are many other lung

Table 2.2 One method of coding a three category variable.

Status	x_1	x_2	x_3
Children with asthma	1	0	0
Children with bronchitis	0	1	0
Children without either	0	0	1

diseases they might have. In this table the categories are mutually exclusive (i.e. there are no children with both asthma and bronchitis). Table 2.2 gives possible dummy variables for a group of three subjects.

A possible model is:

$$\text{Deadspace} = \beta_0 + \beta_{\text{Asthma}} \times \text{Asthma} + \beta_{\text{Bronchitis}} \times \text{Bronchitis} \tag{2.6}$$

We now have three possible contrasts: children with asthma vs children with bronchitis, children with asthma vs children without asthma or bronchitis and children with bronchitis vs children without asthma or bronchitis, but they are not all independent. Knowing two of the contrasts we can deduce the third (if you do not have asthma or bronchitis, then you *must* be normal). Thus we need to choose two of the three contrasts to include in the regression and thus two dummy variables to include in the regression. It is important to note that including bronchitis in the model changes the interpretation of the asthma coefficient (β_{Asthma}). Without it, the asthma coefficient is the comparison between children with and without asthma, and the latter category includes those with bronchitis. Including the bronchitis dummy in the model means that the comparison is between children without either asthma or bronchitis. If we included all three variables in a regression, most programs would inform us politely that x_1, x_2 and x_3 were *aliased* (i.e. mutually dependent) and omit one of the variables from the equation. The dummy variable that is omitted from the regression is the one that the coefficients for the other variables are contrasted with, and is known as the *baseline* variable. Thus if x_3 is omitted in the regression that includes x_1 and x_2 in Table 2.2, then the coefficient attached to x_1 is the difference between deadspace for children with and without asthma. Another way of looking at it is that the coefficient associated with the baseline (normal) is constrained to be 0.

2.4 Interpreting a Computer Output

We now describe how to interpret a computer output for linear regression. Most statistical packages produce an output similar to this one. The models are fitted using the *principle of least squares*, as explained in Appendix 2, and is equivalent to maximum likelihood when the error distribution is Normal. The estimate of the standard error (SE) is more sensitive to the Normality assumption than the estimate of the coefficients. There are two options available which do not require this assumption; these are the *bootstrap* and the *robust standard error*. These are available in R and are described in Appendix 3.

2.4.1 One Continuous Variable

The results of fitting model 2.2 to the data are shown in Table 2.3.

The computer program gives three sections of output.

The first part gives the distribution of the residuals, that is, estimates of the ε_i from the model. The minimum, first quartile, median, third quartile and maximum are given. The model will force the mean of the residuals to be zero and if the distribution of the residuals is symmetric we would expect the median to be close to zero as well, and in this case that is so. It is also a good idea to check that the minimum and maximum are not too extreme, which in this case they are not.

The second part examines the coefficients in the model. The slope $\beta_{Height} = 1.0333$ ml/cm and suggests that if one person was 1 cm taller than another we would expect their deadspace to be about 1 ml greater (perhaps easier to think that if one person were 10 cm taller their deadspace is expected to be 10 ml greater). It is the slope of the line in Figure 2.1. The intercept is $\beta_0 = -82.4852$. This is the value when the line cuts the y-axis when $x = 0$ (not the axis on the figure which is at $x = 110$). This is the predicted value of deadspace for someone with no height and is clearly a nonsense value and the test of significance should not be quoted in publications. However, the parameter is necessary for correct interpretation of the model. Note these values are derived directly in Chapter 9 of *Statistics at Square One.*

The third part refers to fit of the overall model. The $F = 32.81$ is what is known as an F-statistic (after the statistician RA Fisher), which depends on two numbers known as the *degrees of freedom*. The first, p, is the number of parameters in the model (excluding the constant term β_0), which in this case is 1 and the second is $n - p - 1$, where n is the number

Table 2.3 Output from computer program fitting height to deadspace for data from Table 2.1.

```
Residuals:
     Min       1Q   Median       3Q      Max
-17.8132  -6.8135  -0.7132   8.2533  20.8869

Coefficients:
            Estimate Std. Error t value Pr(>|t|)
(Intercept) -82.4852    26.3015  -3.136  0.00788
Height        1.0333     0.1804   5.728 6.96e-05

Residual standard error: 13.07 on 13 degrees of freedom
Multiple R-squared:  0.7162,    Adjusted R-squared:  0.6944
F-statistic: 32.81 on 1 and 13 DF, p-value: 6.956e-05

# Confidence intervals
                   2.5%      97.5%
(Intercept) -139.3060636 -25.664333
Height         0.6436202   1.423026
```

of observations and in this case is 15 – 1 – 1 = 13. The p-value is the probability that the variability associated with the model could have occurred by chance, on the assumption that the true model has only a constant term and no explanatory variables; in other words the overall significance of the model. This is given as 6.956e – 05, that is, 6.956×10^{-5} or 0.00006956. This is better given as $p < 0.001$ since it is spurious to give accuracy to such a small number.

An important statistic is the value R^2 (Multiple R-squared), which is the proportion of variance of the original data explained by the model and in this model it is 0.7162. For models with only one independent variable, as in this case, it is simply the square of the correlation coefficient described in *Statistics at Square One*. However, one can always obtain an arbitrarily good fit by fitting as many parameters as there are observations. To allow for this, we calculate the R^2 *adjusted for degrees of freedom*, which is $R^2_a = 1 - (1 - R^2)(n - 1)/(n - p - 1)$ and in this case (n = 15, p = 1) is given by 0.6944. The Residual SE is an estimate of σ in Equation 2.1 and has the value 13.07. We would like this as small as possible.

Finally, we can easily obtain the 95% confidence interval (CI) for β_{Height}. This is given as 0.64 to 1.42. Thus, our best estimate of the slope is 1.03 ml/cm, but it could be as small as 0.64 ml/cm or as large as 1.42 ml/cm. This is a wide interval because the data set is small.

2.4.2 One Continuous Variable and One Binary Independent Variable

This analysis is often used to compare the outcome variable at different levels of the binary variable, adjusting for the continuous independent variable. It is often called *analysis of covariance*. We must first create a new variable Asthma = 1 for children with asthma and Asthma = 0 for children without asthma. This gives model 2.3 and the results of fitting this model are shown in Table 2.4.

We can see that the residuals have changed somewhat, but the median is still close to zero.

In the middle part of the output, the coefficient associated with height is $\beta_{Height} = 0.845$, which is less than the same coefficient in Table 2.3. It is the slope of each of the parallel lines in Figure 2.2. It can be seen that because children without asthma have a higher deadspace, forcing a single line through the data gives a greater slope. The vertical distance between the two lines is the coefficient associated with asthma, $\beta_{Asthma} = -16.81$, with 95% CI −30.00 to −3.63. As we coded asthma as 1 and non-asthma as 0, the negative sign indicates children with asthma have a lower deadspace of 16.81 ml for a given height. This is statistically significant, with a p-value of 0.017. This model assumes this difference is unaffected by height.

In the third part of the output, the *F*-statistic now has 2 and 12 d.f., because we are fitting two independent variables. The *p*-value is given as 2.653 × 10-5, which we interpret as < 0.001. It means that fitting both variables *simultaneously* gives a highly significant fit. It does *not* tell us about individual variables. One can see that the adjusted R^2 is greater and the Residual SE is smaller than that in Table 2.3, indicating a better fitting model than model 2.2. Since the only difference between model 3.2 and model 3.3 is the coefficient associated with asthma and that is statistically significant, we can say that model 3.3 is a statistically significantly better fit. Whether this is a practically important fit depends on whether having a residual SE of 13.07 is better than one of 10.61.

Table 2.4 Results of fitting model 2.3 to the asthma data.

```
Residuals:
    Min       1Q  Median      3Q     Max
-20.733   -7.395   0.111   7.858  16.324

Coefficients:
            Estimate Std. Error t value Pr(>|t|)
(Intercept) -46.2922    25.0168  -1.850 0.089012
Height        0.8450     0.1614   5.236 0.000209
Asthma      -16.8155     6.0531  -2.778 0.016713

Residual standard error: 10.61 on 12 degrees of freedom
Multiple R-squared: 0.8273, Adjusted R-squared: 0.7985
F-statistic: 28.74 on 2 and 12 DF, p-value: 2.653e-05

#Confidence intervals
                   2.5 %    97.5 %
(Intercept) -100.7990584  8.214733
Height         0.4934035  1.196690
Asthma       -30.0041448 -3.626880
```

2.4.3 One Continuous Variable and One Binary Independent Variable with Their Interaction

We now fit an interaction term in the model. In some packages we would need to create a new variable for the interaction, for example, AsthmaHt = Asthma × Height, whereas other packages can do this automatically by fitting a term such as "Asthma*Height" to give model 2.4. We fit three independent variables: Height, Asthma and Height:Asthma on Deadspace. This is equivalent to model 2.4, and is shown in Figure 2.3. The results of fitting these variables using a computer program are given in Table 2.5.

Now $F(3,11) = 37.08$ and $R^2 = 0.91$, the R^2 adjusted for d.f. is given by 0.89 which is an improvement on model 2.3. The residual SE has the value 8.003, which again indicates an improvement on the earlier model.

In the second part of the output we see that the interaction term between height and asthma status is significant ($P = 0.009$). The *difference* in the slopes is −0.778 units (95% CI −1.317 to −0.240). Note, even if one of the main terms, asthma or height was not significant, we would *not* drop it from the model if the interaction was significant, since the interaction cannot be interpreted in the absence of the main effects, which in this case are asthma and height.

The two lines of best fit are:

Children without asthma:

$$\text{Deadspace} = -99.46 + 1.193 \times \text{Height}$$

Table 2.5 Results of fitting model 2.4 to the asthma data.

```
Residuals:
   Min      1Q Median     3Q    Max
-8.578 -5.750 -1.401  4.065 13.889

Coefficients:
              Estimate Std. Error t value Pr(>|t|)
(Intercept)   -99.4624    25.2079  -3.946  0.00229
Height          1.1926     0.1636   7.291 1.56e-05
Asthma         95.4726    35.6106   2.681  0.02137
Height:Asthma  -0.7782     0.2448  -3.179  0.00877

Residual standard error: 8.003 on 11 degrees of freedom
Multiple R-squared:  0.91,   Adjusted R-squared:  0.8855
F-statistic: 37.08 on 3 and 11 DF,   p-value: 4.803e-06

# Confidence intervals
                      2.5 %     97.5 %
(Intercept)    -154.9447221 -43.980090
Height            0.8325555   1.552574
Asthma1          17.0943233 173.850939
Height:Asthma1   -1.3169959  -0.239503
```

Children with asthma:

$$\text{Deadspace} = (-99.46 + 95.47) + (1.193 - 0.778) \times \text{Height}$$

$$= -3.99 + 0.415 \times \text{Height}$$

Thus, the deadspace in children with asthma appears to grow more slowly with height than that of children without asthma.

This is the best fit model for the data so far investigated. Using model 2.2 or 2.3 for prediction, say, would result in a greater error. It is important, when considering which is the best model, to look at the R^2 adjusted as well as the p-values. Sometimes a term can be added that gives a significant p-value, but only a marginal improvement in R^2 adjusted, and for the sake of simplicity may not be included as the best model.

2.4.4 Two Independent Variables: Both Continuous

Here we were interested in whether height or age or both were important in the prediction of deadspace. The analysis is given in Table 2.6.

The equation is:

$$\text{Deadspace} = -59.05 + 0.707 \times \text{Height} + 3.045 \times \text{Age}$$

Table 2.6 Results of fitting model 2.5 to the asthma data.

```
Residuals:
    Min      1Q  Median      3Q     Max
-15.481  -7.827  -2.615   7.749  22.213

Coefficients:
            Estimate Std. Error t value Pr(>|t|)
(Intercept) -59.0520    33.6316  -1.756   0.1046
Height        0.7070     0.3455   2.046   0.0633
Age           3.0447     2.7585   1.104   0.2913
---
Residual standard error: 12.96 on 12 degrees of freedom
Multiple R-squared:  0.7424,   Adjusted R-squared:  0.6995
F-statistic: 17.29 on 2 and 12 DF,  p-value: 0.0002922

#95% Confidence intervals
                    2.5 %    97.5 %
(Intercept) -132.32904832 14.224952
Height        -0.04582684  1.459890
Age           -2.96560200  9.054984
```

The interpretation of this model is described in Section 2.3.2. Note a peculiar feature of this output. Although the overall model is significant ($P = 0.0003$) neither of the coefficients associated with height and age are significant ($P = 0.063$ and 0.291, respectively). This occurs because age and height are strongly correlated (despite being called "independent variables"), and highlights the importance of looking at the overall fit of a model. Dropping either will leave the other as a significant predictor in the model. Note that if we drop age, the adjusted R^2 is not greatly affected ($R^2 = 0.6944$ for height alone compared to 0.6995 for age and height) suggesting that height is a better predictor. One way of investigating this is using the standardised coefficients given in Table 2.7. In this case, the intercept is the standardised deadspace predicted by the mean height and mean age, which is zero since the regression line is constrained to go through both means. This is perhaps more sensible than that of Table 2.6 which predicts the deadspace for age and height zero. The coefficients are now comparable, since both age and height are standardised to have mean zero and s.d. one. One can see that height has approximately twice the size of age. As one might expect, since standardised age and height are simple scaled age and height, the t-statistics and p-values are exactly the same as in Table 2.7.

It is possible to plot the model with two continuous independent variables in a so-called "3D plot" where the fitted values on the y-axis are depicted as a plane, with one independent variable as the x-axis and the other apparently going into the page, but it is of limited value. An alternative 2D plot is to plot y against x_1 for fixed values of x_2.

Table 2.7 Results using age and height standardised to have mean zero and s.d. one.

```
Standardised Coefficients:
               Estimate  Std. Error  t value Pr(>|t|)
(Intercept) -2.826e-16   1.415e-01    0.000    1.0000
Heightstd    5.791e-01   2.830e-01    2.046    0.0633.
Agestd       3.124e-01   2.830e-01    1.104    0.2913
```

2.4.5 Categorical Independent Variables

Here, the two independent variables are asthma and bronchitis. It will help the interpretation in this section to know that the mean values (ml) for deadspace for the three groups are: children without asthma or bronchitis 97.33, children with asthma 52.88 and children with bronchitis 72.25. The analysis is given in Table 2.8.

As we noted before, an important point to check is that, in general, one should see that the overall model is significant, before looking at the individual contrasts. Here we have p-value 0.006275, which means that the overall model is highly significant, that is, it is better than a simple mean which is what the default model is. If we look at the individual

Table 2.8 Results of fitting asthma and bronchitis to deadspace.

```
# Asthma and Bronchitis as independent variables

Residuals:
     Min       1Q  Median       3Q      Max
 -41.250   -8.375   3.667    8.438   19.750

 Coefficients:
              Estimate Std. Error t value Pr(>|t|)
 (Intercept)    97.333      9.664  10.072 3.32e-07
 Asthma        -44.458     11.332  -3.923  0.00202
 Bronchitis    -25.083     12.785  -1.962  0.07338 .
 ---

 Residual standard error: 16.74 on 12 degrees of freedom
 Multiple R-squared: 0.5705, Adjusted R-squared: 0.499
 F-statistic: 7.971 on 2 and 12 DF,  p-value: 0.006275

# Confidence intervals
                  2.5 %      97.5 %
Intercept      76.27682   118.38984
Asthma        -69.14928   -19.76739
Bronchitis    -52.93848     2.77181
```

contrasts, we see that the coefficient associated with asthma −44.46 is the difference in means between children with asthma and children without asthma or bronchitis. This has a SE of 11.33 and so is highly significant. The coefficient associated with being bronchitic is −25.08; the contrast between children with bronchitis and children without asthma or bronchitis is not significant, implying that the mean deadspace is not significantly different in children with bronchitis and children without asthma or bronchitis. Note, this doesn't mean that there is no difference between children with bronchitis and children without asthma or bronchitis, simply that the sample is relatively small and so we do not have enough numbers to demonstrate a conclusive difference.

If we wished to contrast children with asthma from children with bronchitis, we would need to make one of them the baseline. Thus we make asthma and normal the independent variables, to make children with bronchitis the baseline and the output is shown in the Table 2.9.

As would be expected, the p-value and the R^2 value are the same as the earlier model because these refer to the overall model which differs from the earlier one only in the formulation of the parameters. However, now the coefficients refer to the contrast with bronchitis and we can see that the difference between children with asthma and bronchitis has a difference −19.38 with SE 10.25, which is not significant. Thus, the only significant difference is between children with and without asthma.

This method of analysis is also known as *one-way analysis of variance*. It is a generalisation of the *t*-test referred to in Campbell.[1] One could ask what is the difference between this

Table 2.9 Results of fitting asthma and normal to deadspace.

```
# Asthma and Normal as independent variables

Residuals:
     Min       1Q  Median       3Q      Max
 -41.250   -8.375   3.667    8.438   19.750

 Coefficients:
              Estimate  Std. Error  t value  Pr(>|t|)
 Intercept      72.250       8.369    8.633  1.71e-06
 Asthma        -19.375      10.250   -1.890    0.0831
 Normal         25.083      12.785    1.962    0.0734
---

Residual standard error: 16.74 on 12 degrees of freedom
Multiple R-squared: 0.5705, Adjusted R-squared: 0.499
F-statistic: 7.971 on 2 and 12 DF, p-value: 0.006275

# Confidence intervals
                    2.5 %     97.5 %
(Intercept)      54.01453   90.48547
Asthma          -41.70880    2.95880
Normal           -2.77181   52.93848
```

and simply carrying out two t tests: children with asthma vs children without asthma and children with bronchitis vs children without bronchitis. In fact, the analysis of variance accomplishes two extra refinements. First, the overall p-value controls for the problem of multiple testing. By doing a number of tests against the baseline we are increasing the chances of a Type I error. The overall p-value in the F-test allows for this and since it is significant, we know that some of the contrasts must be significant. The second improvement is that in order to calculate a t-test we must find the pooled SE. In the t-test this is done from two groups, whereas in the analysis of variance it is calculated from all three, which is based on more subjects and so is more precise.

2.5 Examples in the Medical Literature

2.5.1 Analysis of Covariance: One Binary and One Continuous Independent Variable

We mentioned that model 2.3 is very commonly seen in the literature. To see its application in a clinical trial consider the results of Llewellyn-Jones *et al.*,[3] part of which are given in Table 2.10. This study was a randomised-controlled trial of the effectiveness of a shared care intervention for depression in 220 subjects over the age of 65 years. Depression was measured using the Geriatric Depression Scale, taken at baseline and after 9.5 months of blinded follow-up. The figure that helps the interpretation is Figure 2.2. Here, y is the depression scale after 9.5 months of treatment (continuous), x_1 is the value of the same scale at baseline and x_2 is the group variable, taking the value 1 for intervention and 0 for control.

The authors give the *standardised regression coefficients* as well, although in this case they are not particularly helpful. One can see that the baseline values are highly correlated with the follow-up values of the score. The intervention resulted, on average, in patients with a score 1.87 units (95% CI 0.76 to 2.97) lower than those in the control group, throughout the range of the baseline values.

This analysis assumes that the treatment effect is the same for all subjects and is not related to values of their baseline scores. This possibility could be checked by the methods discussed earlier. When two groups are balanced with respect to the baseline value, one might assume that including the baseline value in the analysis will not affect the comparison of treatment groups. However, it is often worthwhile including this because it can improve the precision of the estimate of the treatment effect; that is, the SEs of the treatment effects may be smaller when the baseline covariate is included.

Table 2.10 Factors affecting Geriatric Depression Scale score at follow-up.

Variable	Regression coefficient (95% CI)	Standardised regression coefficient	*P*-value
Baseline score	0.73 (0.56 to 0.91)	0.56	<0.0001
Treatment group	−1.87 (−2.97 to −0.76)	−0.22	0.0011

Llewellyn-Jones RH, Baikie KA, Smithers H, Cohen J, Snowdon J, Tennant CC. Multifaceted shared care intervention for late life depression in residential care: randomised controlled trial. *Br Med J* 1999; **319:** 676–82.

2.5.2 Two Continuous Independent Variables

Sorensen *et al.*[4] describe a cohort study of 4300 men, aged between 18 and 26, who had their body mass index (BMI) measured. The investigators wished to relate adult BMI to the men's birth weight and body length at birth. Potential confounding factors included gestational age, birth order, mother's marital status, age and occupation. In a multiple linear regression they found an association between birth weight (coded in units of 250 g) and BMI (allowing for confounders), regression coefficient 0.82 and SE 0.17, but not between birth length (cm) and BMI, regression coefficient 1.51, SE 3.87. Thus, for every increase in birth weight of 250 g, the BMI increases on average by 0.82kg/m^2. The authors suggest that *in utero* factors that affect birth weight continue to have an affect even into adulthood, even allowing for factors, such as gestational age.

2.6 Assumptions Underlying the Models

There are a number of assumptions implicit in the choice of the model. The most fundamental assumption is that the model is *linear*. This means that each increase by one unit of an x variable is associated by a fixed increase in the y variable, irrespective of the starting value of the x variable.

There are a number of ways of checking this when x is continuous:

- For single continuous independent variables the simplest check is a visual one from a scatter plot of y vs x.
- Try transformations of the x variables ($\log x$, x^2 and $1/x$ are the commonest). There is not a simple significance test for one transformation against another, but a good guide would be if the R^2 value gets larger.
- Include a quadratic term (x^2) as well as the linear term (x) in the model. This model is the one where we fit two continuous variables, x and x^2. A significant coefficient for x^2 indicates a lack of linearity.
- Divide x into a number groups such as by quintiles. Fit separate dummy variables for the four largest quintile groups and examine the coefficients. For a linear relationship, the coefficients themselves will increase linearly.

Another fundamental assumption is that the error terms are independent of each other. An example of where this is unlikely is when the data form a time series. A simple check for sequential data for independent errors is whether the residuals are correlated, and a test known as the *Durbin–Watson* test is available in many packages. Further details are given in Chapter 8, on time series analysis. A further example of lack of independence is where the main unit of measurement is the individual, but several observations are made on each individual, and these are treated as if they came from different individuals. This is the problem of *repeated measures*. A similar type of problem occurs when groups of patients are randomised, rather than individual patients. These are discussed in Chapter 5, on repeated measures.

The model also assumes that the error terms are independent of the x variables and variance of the error term is constant (the latter goes under the more complicated term of *heteroscedascity*). A common alternative is when the error increases as one of the x variables increases, so one way of checking this assumption would be to plot the residuals e_i against each of the independent variables and also against the fitted values. If the model was correct one would expect to see the scatter of residuals evenly spread about the horizontal axis and not showing any pattern. A common departure from this is when the residuals fan out; that is, the scatter gets larger as the x variable gets larger. This is often also associated with non-linearity as well, and so attempts at transforming the x variable may resolve this issue.

The final assumption is that the error term is Normally distributed. One could check this by plotting a histogram of the residuals, although the method of fitting will mean that the observed residuals e_i are likely to be closer to a Normal distribution than the true ones ε_i. The assumption of Normality is important mainly so that we can use Normal theory to estimate CIs around the coefficients, but luckily with reasonably large sample sizes, the estimation method is robust to departures from Normality. Thus, moderate departures from Normality are allowable. If one was concerned, then one could also use bootstrap methods and the robust SE described in Appendix 3.

It is important to remember that the main purpose of this analysis is to assess a relationship, *not* test assumptions, so often we can come to a useful conclusion *even when the assumptions are not perfectly satisfied.*

2.7 Model Sensitivity

Model sensitivity refers to how estimates are affected by subgroups of the data. Suppose we had fitted a simple regression (model 2.2), and we were told that the estimates b_0 and b_1 altered dramatically if you delete a subset of the data, or even a single individual. This is important, because we like to think that the model applies generally, and we do not wish to find that we should have different models for different subgroups of patients.

2.7.1 Residuals, Leverage and Influence

There are three main issues in identifying model sensitivity to individual observations: *residuals, leverage* and *influence*. The residuals are the difference between the observed and fitted data: $e_i = y_i^{obs} - y_i^{fit}$. A point with a large residual is called an outlier. In general, we are interested in outliers because they may influence the estimates, but it is possible to have a large outlier which is not influential. Outliers are also give clear evidence of data not conforming to the model and decisions have to be made whether to believe the outlier or the model.

Another way that a point can be an outlier is if the values of the x_i are a long way from the mass of x. For a single variable, this means if x_i is a long way from $\bar{x}$. Imagine a scatter plot of y against x, with a mass of points in the bottom-left-hand corner and a single point in the top right. It is possible that this individual has unique characteristics that relate to both the x and y variables. A regression line fitted to the data will go close, or even through the isolated point. This isolated point will not have a large residual, yet if this point is deleted the regression coefficient might change dramatically. Such a point is said to have high *leverage* and this can be measured by a number, often denoted h_i; large values of h_i indicate a high leverage.

An influential point is one that has a large effect on an estimate. Effectively one fits the model with and without that point and finds the effect of the regression coefficient. One might look for points that have a large effect on b_0, or on b_1 or on other estimates such as

SE(b_1). The usual output is the difference in the regression coefficient for a particular variable when the point is included or excluded, scaled by the estimated SE of the coefficient. The problem is that different parameters may have different influential points. Most computer packages now produce residuals, leverages and influential points as a matter of routine. It is the task for an analyst to examine these and to identify important cases. However, just because a case is influential or has a large residual it does not follow that it should be deleted, although the data should be examined carefully for possible measurement or transcription errors. A proper analysis of such data would report such sensitivities to individual points.

2.7.2 Computer Analysis: Model Checking and Sensitivity

We will illustrate model checking and sensitivity using the deadspace, age and height data in Table 2.1.

Figure 2.1 gives us reassurance that the relationship between deadspace and height is plausibly linear. We could plot a similar graph for deadspace and age. The standard diagnostic plot is a plot of the residuals against the fitted values, and for the model fitted in Table 2.6 it is shown in Figure 2.4. There is no apparent pattern, which gives us reassurance about the error term being relatively constant and further reassurance about the linearity of the model.

The diagnostic statistics are shown in Table 2.11, where the *influence* statistics are *inf_age* associated with age and *inf_ht* associated with height. As one might, expect the children with the highest leverages are the youngest (who is also the shortest) and the oldest (who is also the tallest). Note that the largest residuals are associated with small leverages. This is because points with large leverage will tend to force the line close to them.

The child with the most influence on the age coefficient is also the oldest, and removal of that child would change the standardised regression coefficient by 0.79 units. The child with the most influence on height is the shortest child.

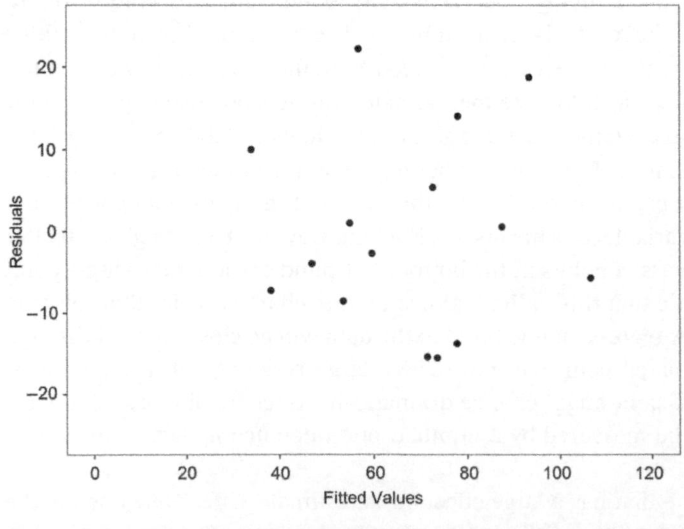

Figure 2.4 Graph of residuals against fitted values for model 2.6 using age and height as independent variables.

Table 2.11 Diagnostics from model fitted in Table 2.4 (output from computer program).

	Height	Age	Resids	Leverage	inf_age	inf_ht
1	110	5	10.06	0.33	0.22	−0.48
2	116	5	−7.19	0.23	−0.04	0.18
3	124	6	−3.89	0.15	−0.03	0.08
4	129	7	−8.47	0.15	−0.14	0.20
5	131	7	1.12	0.12	0.01	−0.02
6	138	6	22.21	0.13	−0.52	0.34
7	142	6	−2.61	0.17	0.08	−0.06
8	150	8	−15.36	0.08	0.11	−0.14
9	153	8	−15.48	0.10	0.20	−0.26
10	155	9	14.06	0.09	0.02	0.07
11	156	7	5.44	0.28	−0.24	0.25
12	159	8	−13.72	0.19	0.38	−0.46
13	164	10	0.65	0.14	0.00	0.01
14	168	11	18.78	0.19	0.29	0.08
15	174	14	−5.60	0.65	−0.79	0.42

However, neither child should be removed without strong reason. (A strong reason may be if it was discovered the child had some relevant disease, such as cystic fibrosis.)

2.8 Stepwise Regression

When one has a large number of independent variables, a natural question to ask is what is the best combination of these variables to predict the y variable? To answer this, one may use *stepwise* regression that is available in a number of packages. *Step-down* or *backwards* regression starts by fitting all available variables and then discarding sequentially those that are not significant. *Step-up* or *forwards* regression starts by fitting an overall mean, and then selecting variables to add to the model according to their significance. *Stepwise* regression is a mixture of the two, where one can specify *p*-value for a variable to be entered into the model, and then a *p*-value for a variable to be discarded. Usually one chooses a larger *p*-value for entry (say, 0.1) than for exclusion (say, 0.05), since variables can jointly be predictive and separately they are not. This also favours *step-down* regression. As an example, consider an outcome variable being the amount a person limps. The length of the left or right legs is not predictive, but the difference in lengths is highly predictive. Stepwise regression is best used in the *exploratory* phase of an analysis (see Chapter 1), to identify a few predictors in a mass of data, the association of which can be verified by further data collection.

There are a few problems with stepwise regression:

- The *p*-values are invalid since they do not take account of the vast number of tests that have been carried out; different methods, such as step-up and step-down are likely to

produce different models and experience shows that the same model rarely emerges when a second data set is analysed. One way of trying to counter this is to split a large data set into two and run the stepwise procedure on both separately. Choose the variables that are common to both data sets, and fit these to the combined data sets as the final model.
- Many large data sets contain missing values. With stepwise regression, usually only the subjects who have no missing values on *any* of the variables under consideration are chosen. The final model may contain only a few variables, but if one refits the model, the parameters change because now the model is being fitted to those subjects who have no missing values on only the few chosen variables, which may be a considerably larger data set than the original.
- If a categorical variable is coded as a number of dummies, some of these may be lost in the fitting process and this changes the interpretation of the others. Thus, if we fitted x_1 and x_2 from Table 2.2, and then we lost x_2, the interpretation of x_1 is of a contrast between children with asthma with children with bronchitis and children without asthma or bronchitis *combined.*

2.9 Reporting the Results of a Multiple Regression

- As a minimum, report the regression coefficients and SEs or CIs for the main independent variables, together with the adjusted R^2 for the whole model.
- If there is one main dependent variable, show a scatter plot of each independent variable vs dependent variable with the best-fit line.
- Report how the assumptions underlying the model were tested and verified. In particular, is linearity plausible?
- Report any sensitivity analysis carried out.
- Report any tests of interactions.
- Report *all* the variables included in the model. For a stepwise regression, report *all* the variables that could have entered the model.
- Note that if an interaction term is included in a model, the main effects *must* be included.
- Report how missing values were treated in the analysis.
- If relevant, report how outlying data were treated.
- Try and show the data graphically.

Further considerations are given in the SAMPL and CHAMPS checklists.[5,6]

2.10 Reading about the Results of a Multiple Regression

In addition to the points in Section 1.11:

- Note the value of R^2. With a large study, the coefficients in the model can be highly significant, but only explain a low proportion of the variability of the outcome variable. Thus, they may be of no use for prediction.

- Are the models plausibly linear? Are there any boundaries which may cause the slope to flatten?
- Were outliers and influential points identified and how were they treated?
- An analysis of covariance *assumes* that the slopes are the same in each group. Is this plausible and has it been tested?

2.11 Frequently Asked Questions

1) *Does it matter how a dummy variable is coded?*
   If you have only one binary variable, then coding the dummy variable 0 and 1 is the most convenient. Coding it 1 and 2 is commonly the method in questionnaires. It will make no difference to the coefficient estimate or p-value. However it will change the value of the intercept, because now the value in the group assigned 1 will be $a + b$ and the value in the group assigned 2 will be $a + 2b$. Thus, in Figure 2.2 when "Asthma" is coded 0 the intercept is −46.29. If we had coded "Asthma" 1 for non-asthma then the intercept has to be $(-46.3 - -16.8) = -29.5$. Coding the dummy variable to −1 and +1 (as is done, for example in the package SAS) does not change the p-value but the coefficient is halved.

   If you have a categorical variable with, say, three groups, then this will be coded with two dummy variables. As shown earlier, the overall *F*-statistic will be unchanged no matter which two groups are chosen to be represented by dummies, but the coefficient of group 2, say, will depend on whether group 1 or group 3 is the omitted variable.
2) *How do I treat an ordinal independent variable?*
   Most packages assume that the predictor variable, *X*, in a regression model is either continuous or binary. Thus, one has a number of options.

   a) Treat the predictor as if it were continuous. This incorporates into the model the fact that the categories are ordered, but also assumes that equal changes in *X* mean equal changes in *y*.
   b) Treat the predictor as if it were categorical by fitting dummy variables to all but one of the categories. This loses the fact that the predictor is ordinal, but makes no assumption about linearity.
   c) Dichotomise the *X* variable, by recoding it as binary, say 1 if X is in a particular category or above, and zero otherwise. The cut point should be chosen on external grounds and not because it gives the best fit to the data.

   Which of these options is chosen depends on a number of factors. With a large amount of data, the loss of information by ignoring the ordinality in option 2 is not critical, especially if the *X* variable is a confounder and not of prime interest. For example, if *X* is age grouped in ten-year intervals, it might be better to fit dummy variables than assume a linear relation with the y variable.
3) *Do the assumptions underlying multiple regression matter?*
   Often the assumptions underlying multiple regression are not checked, partly because the investigator is confident that they hold true and partly because mild departures

are unlikely to invalidate an analysis. However, lack of independence may be obvious on empirical grounds (the data form repeated measures or a time series) and so the analysis should accommodate this from the outset. Linearity is important for inference and so may be checked by fitting transformations of the independent variables. Lack of homogeneity of variance and lack of Normality may affect the SEs and often indicate the need for a transformation of the dependent variable. The most common departure from Normality is when outliers are identified, and these should be carefully checked, particularly those with high leverage.

4) *I have a variable that I believe should be a confounder but it is not significant. Should I include it in the analysis?*
There are certain variables (such as age or sex) for which one might have strong grounds for believing that they could be confounders, but in any particular analysis may emerge as significant. These should be retained in the analysis because, even if not significantly related to the outcome themselves, they may modify the effect of the prime independent variable.
5) *What happens if I have a dependent variable which is 0 or 1?*
When the dependent variable is 0 or 1 then the coefficients from a linear regression are proportional to what is known as the *linear discriminant function*. This can be useful for discriminating between groups, even if the assumption about Normality of the residuals is violated. However, discrimination is normally carried out now using *logistic regression* (Chapter 3).

2.12 Exercises: Reading the Literature

Exercise 2.1

Melchart *et al.*[7] describe a randomised trial of acupuncture in 205 patients with tension-type headache with 2:1 randomisation to either acupuncture for eight weeks or a waiting list control. Partial results are given in the Table 2.12.

Using a t-test on the difference in outcome from baseline to after treatment the authors found a difference between groups of 5.7 days (95% CI 4.2 to 7.2) $P < 0.001$. The authors then conducted an analysis of covariance on the outcome variables, adjusting for baseline value. They found the difference between groups after treatment: 5.8 days (95% CI 4.0 to 7.6) $P < 0.001$.

a) Give three assumptions made for the analysis of covariance.
b) What evidence do we have that these may not be satisfied?
c) Contrast the two CIs.
d) What other plots of the data might one like to see?
e) Why did the adjustment for baseline matter so little?

Exercise 2.2

Bélanger-Lévesque and colleagues[8] conducted a cross-sectional study of 200 mothers and 200 accompanying partners 12–24 hours after the birth over a six-week period. The outcome was the Birth Satisfaction Scale (BSS) and they used multiple linear regression

Table 2.12 Results from the Melchart *et al.*[7] trial of 205 people for acupuncture in headache.

	Acupuncture	Waiting list
Baseline	17.5 (6.9) ($n = 132$)	17.3 (6.9) ($n = 75$)
After treatment	9.9 (8.7) ($n = 118$)	16.3 (7.4) ($n = 63$)

Values are represented as days with headache during a 28-day period (Mean (SD)). Data from [7].

Table 2.13 Delivery factors influencing satisfaction with birth (vaginal deliveries).

	Non-standardised coefficients		Standardised coefficients			Model		
Variable	B	SE(B)	β	t	p-value	F	p-value	Adjusted R^2
Epidural (yes)	−6.99	1.85	−0.30	−3.74	0.000			
Peri-urethral tear	4.37	1.72	0.19	2.54	0.012	4.07	0.045	0.194
Labour length (Total)	−0.01	0.01	−0.18	−2.20	0.029			
Perineal tear third degree	−7.29	3.62	−0.15	−2.02	0.045			

Omitted variables: No anaesthesia, first stage labour length, second stage labour length, instrumental birth.

to assess factors of the delivery which were associated with satisfaction. A higher score on the BSS indicates a higher satisfaction. Factors include six types of anaesthesia (including none), and three degrees of perineal tear. For the 157 women who had a vaginal delivery, initially they used regression with single covariates to find which factors were significantly associated with the BSS. Those that were significant were put in a stepwise model and four who were jointly non-significant were excluded. The results are given in Table 2.13. Consider the points in Sections 2.10 and 2.11 and answer the following questions.

a) Describe the effect of the delivery factors on the BSS satisfaction score. Are there any surprises?
b) What does the p-value for the model test?
c) What do the standardised coefficients tell the reader?
d) What assumption is made about total labour length?
e) What issues are there with using categorical variables such as Epidural in a step-wise regression?
f) What is the reference that the perineal tear third degree coefficient is compared to?
g) Do the length of first stage and second stage labour not matter, since the stepwise regression threw them out?
h) Does the model do a good job in explaining satisfaction?

References

1 Campbell MJ. *Statistics at Square One*, 12th edn. Chichester: Wiley, 2021.

2 Draper NR, Smith H. *Applied Regression Analysis*, 3rd edn. New York: John Wiley, 1998.

3 Llewellyn-Jones RH, Baikie KA, Smithers H, Cohen J, Snowdon J, Tennant CC. Multifaceted shared care intervention for late life depression in residential care: randomised controlled trial. *Br Med J* 1999; **319**: 676–82.

4 Sorensen HT, Sabroe S, Rothman KJ, Gillman M, Fischer P, Sorensen TIA. Relation between weight and length at birth and body mass index in young adulthood: cohort study. *Br Med J* 1997; **315**: 1137.

5 Lang TA, Altman DG. Basic statistical reporting for articles published in biomedical journals: the "statistical analyses and methods in the published literature" or the SAMPL guidelines. *Int J Nurs Stud.* 2015; **52**(1): 5–9.

6 Mansournia MA, Collins GS, Nielsen RO, *et al.* A checklist for statistical assessment of medical papers (the CHAMP statement): explanation and elaboration. *Br J Sports Med.* 2021; **55**: 1009–1017. doi: 10.1136/bjsports-2020-103652

7 Melchart D, Streng A, Hoppe A, Brinkhaus B, Witt C, *et al.* Acupuncture in patients with tension-type headache: randomised controlled trial. *Br Med J* 2005; **331**: 376–82.

8 Bélanger-Lévesque M-N, Pasquier M, Roy-Matton N, *et al.* Maternal and paternal satisfaction in the delivery room: a cross-sectional comparative study. *BMJ Open* 2014; **4**: e004013. doi: 10.1136/bmjopen-2013-004013

3

Multiple Logistic Regression

Summary

The chi-squared test is used for testing the association between two binary variables. Logistic regression is a generalisation of linear regression to examine the association of a binary dependent variable with one or more independent variables that can be binary, categorical (more than two categories) or continuous. It can test the same hypothesis as the chi-squared test but does much more, such as giving estimates of measures of association and confidence intervals (CI). It is often used to develop predictive models. Logistic regression is particularly useful for analysing *case-control* studies. Matched case-control studies require a particular analysis known as *conditional logistic regression*.

3.1 Quick Revision

Chapters 4 and 10 in *Statistics at Square One* describe the handling of binary data. Here we give a quick revision to establish the definitions. For a binary dependent variable, the outcome can be described as an *event* which is either present or absent (sometimes termed "success" or "failure"). Thus, an event might be the presence of a disease in a survey or cure from disease in a clinical trial. We wish to examine factors associated with the event. Since we can rarely predict exactly whether an event will happen or not, what we in fact look for are factors associated with the *probability* of an event happening. Given two binary variables, one of which is the outcome and one of which is a predictor, we can code them both as 1 and 0 and the results are summarised in a 2 × 2 table, Table 3.1.

The Relative Risk (RR) of an event, given the presence of a predictor is:

$$RR = \frac{p_1}{p_0} = \frac{a/(a+b)}{c/(c+d)} = \frac{a(c+d)}{c(a+b)} \tag{3.1}$$

where p_1 and p_0 are the proportion of events when the predictor variable is 1 or 0 respectively.

Statistics at Square Two: Understanding Modern Statistical Application in Medicine, Third Edition.
Michael J. Campbell and Richard M. Jacques.

Table 3.1 A typical 2 × 2 table.

		Outcome		
		Event = 1	Event = 0	Total
Predictor variable	1 = Present	a	b	a + b
	0 = Absent	c	d	c + d
	Total	a + c	b + d	N

The odds of an outcome, given the predictor is present, is: $o_1 = a/b$, and the odds of an event, given the predictor is absent, is: $o_0 = c/d$. So $p_1 = o_1/(1 + o_1)$ and similarly with p_0.

The Odds Ratio (OR) of an event, given the presence of a predictor is:

$$OR = \frac{p_1/(1-p_1)}{p_0/(1-p_0)} = \frac{o_1}{o_0} = \frac{a/b}{c/d} = \frac{ad}{bc} \tag{3.2}$$

When the outcome is quite uncommon, and so a and c are small, the RR and the OR are similar.

For a case-control study, where the outcome is whether a person is a case or a control, the RR estimate is meaningless and we can only estimate the OR. The rare disease assumption means that when the disease is uncommon, we can use the OR from a case-control study to estimate the RR. This is explained in *Statistics at Square One* Chapter 4.

3.2 The Model

As discussed in Chapter 1, writing a model for the analysis is a much more flexible method of analysing data and a more precise way of clarifying assumptions than simply a test. There are two situations to be considered when the outcome is binary:

1) When all the independent variables are categorical and so one can form tables in which each cell has individuals with the same values as the independent variables. As a consequence one can calculate the proportion of subjects for whom an event happens. For example, one might wish to examine the presence or absence of a disease by gender (two categories) and social class (five categories). Thus, one could form a table with the ten social class-by-gender categories and examine the proportion of subjects with disease in each grouping.
2) When the data table contains as many cells as there are individuals and the observed proportions of subjects with disease in each cell must be 0 out of 1 or 1 out of 1. This can occur when at least one of the independent variables is continuous, but of course can also be simply a consequence of the way the data are input. It is possible that each individual has a unique set of predictors and we may not wish to group them.

The purpose of statistical analysis is to take *samples* to estimate *population* parameters (see *Statistics at Square One*). In logistic regression we model the population parameters. If we consider the categorical-grouped case first, denote the population probability of an event for a cell i by π_i. This is also called the "expected" value. Thus, for an unbiased coin the population or expected probability for a "head" is 0.5. The dependent variable, p_i, is the observed proportion of events in the cell (say, the proportion of heads in a set of tosses) and we write $E(p_i) = \pi_i$ where E denotes "expected value".

The model for logistic regression with p independent variables is:

$$log_e\left(\frac{\pi_i}{1-\pi_i}\right) = logit(\pi_i) = \beta_0 + \beta_1 X_{i1} + \ldots + \beta_p X_{ip} \quad (3.3)$$

where the independent variables are $X_{i1},\ldots, X_{ip}$.

The term on the left-hand side of Equation 3.3 is the log odds of success, and is often called the *logistic* or *logit* transform. The terms on the right-hand side can be binary, categorical or continuous.

The reason why model 3.3 is useful is that the coefficients β_i are related to the OR in 2×2 tables. Suppose we had only one independent variable (covariate) X, which was binary and simply takes the values 0 or 1. Then the OR associated with X and the outcome is given by $\exp(\beta)$, note *not* the "RR" as is sometimes stated. If X is continuous, then $\exp(\beta)$ is the OR of an event associated with a unit increase in X.

The main justification for the logit transformation is that the OR is a natural parameter to use for binary outcomes, and the logit transformation relates this to the independent variables in a convenient manner. It can also be justified as follows. The right-hand side of Equation 3.3 is potentially unbounded; that is, can range from minus to plus infinity. On the left-hand side, a probability must lie between 0 and 1. An OR must lie between 0 and infinity. A log OR, or logit, on the other hand, is unbounded and has the same potential range as the right-hand side of Equation 3.3.

Note that at this stage, the *observed* values of the dependent variable are not in the equation. They are linked to the model by the Binomial distribution (described in Appendix 2). Thus, in cell i if we observe y_i successes in n_i subjects, we assume that the y_i are distributed Binomially with probability π_i. The parameters in the model are estimated by maximum likelihood (discussed in Appendix 2). Of course, we do not know the population values π_i, and in the modelling process we substitute into the model the estimated or fitted values.

Often, by analogy to multiple regression, the model is described in the literature as above, but with the observed proportion, $p_i = y_i/n_i$, replacing π_i. This misses out on the second part of a model, the error distribution, that links the two. One could, in fact, use the observed proportions and fit the model by least squares as in multiple regression. In the cases where the 'p_i's are not close to 0 or 1, this will often do well, although the interpretation of the model is different from that of Equation 3.3 as the link with ORs is missing. However, the method of maximum likelihood is easy with current software and is also to be preferred. When the dependent variable is 0/1, the logit of the dependent variable does not exist. This may lead some people to believe that logistic regression is impossible in these circumstances. However, as explained earlier, the model uses the logit of the *expected* value, not the observed value, and the model ensures that the expected value is > 0 and < 1. It can easily be shown that the ungrouped and grouped analyses give exactly the same results in the situations where the covariates are only categorical and so the outcome can be expressed as proportions and not 0/1s.

We may wish to calculate the probability of an event. Suppose we have estimated the coefficients in Equation 3.3 to be b_0, b_1,..., b_p. As in Chapter 1 we write the estimated linear predictor as:

$$\mathrm{LP_i = b_0 + b_1X_{i1} + \ldots + b_pX_{ip}}$$

Then Equation 3.3 can be written as:

$$\hat{\pi}_i = \frac{e^{LP_i}}{1+e^{LP_i}} \tag{3.4}$$

where $\hat{\pi}_i$ is an estimate of π_i and estimates the probability of an event from the model. These are the predicted or fitted values for y_i. A good model will give predictions $\hat{\pi}_i$ close to the observed proportions $p_i = y_i/n_i$.

3.2.1 Categorical Covariates

The Xs in Equation 3.3 are either continuous or binary, as discussed in Chapter 2. To model a categorical or ordinal variable we need to generate a number of so-called "dummy" variables. Suppose we had three nationalities English, Welsh and Scottish. Since there are three groups there are two degrees of freedom (if you are not Welsh or Scottish you must be English (the reference)). These are defined as $X_{Welsh} = 1$ if Welsh, and 0 otherwise and similarly $X_{Scottish} = 1$ if Scottish and 0 otherwise. Any coefficient contrasts one category to the reference, for example X_{Welsh} contrasts the Welsh with the English, ignoring the Scots as long as $X_{Scottish}$ is included in the model. If $X_{Scottish}$ is not included in the model then X_{Welsh} contrasts the English and Scottish combined (much to their annoyance). Similarly, dummy variables can be used for levels of an ordinal variable. It is usual to ignore the fact that an independent ordinal variable has ordinal properties since the loss of precision is usually small. The choice of the "baseline" variable, where the dummy is 0 everywhere, can affect the result. All contrasts are related to this group, so if it is small, the standard error (SE) of the contrast might be high. For this reason it is usual to choose the largest category where the variable is not ordinal. Usually for ordinal variables the baseline is chosen as the lowest (or highest) unless that category is very small.

Further details of logistic regression are given in many books such as Beaumont,[1] Hilbe[2] and Hosmer *et al.*[3]

3.3 Model Checking

There are a number of ways the model may fail to describe the data well. Some of these are the same as those discussed in Section 2.7 for linear regression, such as linearity of the coefficients in the linear predictor, influential observations and lack of an important confounder. Slightly paradoxically, a model in which one of the predictors predicts the outcome perfectly will lead to the model failing to fit since the OR will tend towards infinity.

It is important to look for observations whose removal has a large influence on the model coefficients. These *influential points* are handled in logistic regression in a similar way to that described for multiple regression in Chapter 2, and some computer packages give measures of influence of individual points in logistic regression. These can be checked, and the model refitted omitting them, to see how stable the model is.

Defining residuals and outlying observations is more difficult in logistic regression, when the outcome is 0 or 1, and some parts of model checking are different to the linear regression situation. R gives what are called the deviance residuals which are defined in Appendix 2. Neither Pearson nor deviance residuals are ideal for looking at lack of model fit since they do not follow a Normal distribution and Feng *et al.*[4] suggest "randomised quantile residuals" which introduce an element of randomisation to improve the distribution of the residuals toward Normality. However, this is rarely a critical issue and so is not pursued here.

If a logistic model is to be used for diagnosis or prediction, sometimes a predicted event is defined as happening when $\hat{\pi} > 0.5$ (in fact any value could be used, such as the observed proportion of successes overall). One can then calculate a 2×2 table of actual events versus predicted events to decide if the model is useful. However, this is not commonly done, because a model could identify important risks without being particularly good at predicting them.

Issues particularly pertinent to logistic regression are: lack of fit, "extra-Binomial" variation and the logistic transform.

3.3.1 Lack of Fit

If the independent variables are all categorical, then one can compare the observed proportions in each of the cells and those predicted by the model. However, if some of the input variables are continuous, one has to group the predicted values in some way. Hosmer and Lemeshow[3] suggest a number of methods. One suggestion is to group the predicted probabilities from the model: $\hat{\pi}_i$ and $1-\hat{\pi}_i$ into tenths (by deciles), and compute the predicted number of successes between each decile as the sum of the predicted probabilities for those individuals in that group. Fewer groups may be used if the number of observations is small. The observed number of successes and failures can be compared using a chi-squared distribution with 8 d.f. The reason for there being 8 d.f. is that the basic table has 10 rows and 2 columns (either predicted success or predicted failure) and so 20 initial units. The proportion in each row must add to 1, which gives 10 constraints and the proportion in each column is fixed, to give another 2 constraints and so the number of d.f. is $20 - 10 - 2 = 8$. A well-fitting model should be able to predict the observed successes and failures in each group with some accuracy. A significant chi-squared value indicates that the model is a poor description of the data.

3.3.2 "Extra-binomial" Variation or "Over Dispersion"

Unlike multiple regression, where the size of the residual variance is not specified in advance and is estimated from the data, in logistic regression a consequence of the Binomial model is that the residual variance is predetermined. If we have a series of 0s and 1s with mean π, the variance is given by $\pi(1-\pi)$. If the variance is larger than this it is usually because the assumption that the πs are constant is invalid. This is known as *over-dispersion* or *extra-Binomial variation*. Clearly the πs will vary with the covariates, but when this variation has been allowed for, if the model is reasonable, then the remaining variation should correspond to a Binomial. If this is not the case then the SEs of the parameters may not be well estimated. A simple, ad-hoc method to allow for this is to estimate a dispersion parameter φ which then multiplies the SEs of the parameters of the model, but if it is not incorporated in the model then φ is assumed to be 1. Often over-dispersion occurs when the data are not strictly independent, for example repeated outcomes within an individual, or patients grouped together, such as those treated by the same practitioner. While the estimate of the regression coefficients is not unduly affected, the estimates of the SEs from the model are usually underestimated, leading to CIs that are too narrow. One method of dealing with this is to use SEs that are robust to the assumptions of constant variance, and these are discussed in Appendix 3. Sometimes there is a clear grouping factor and over-dispersion can be accommodated by what is known as a *random effects* model in which one (or more) of the regression coefficients is regarded as random with a mean and variance that can be estimated, rather than fixed. These models are discussed in Chapter 5. A special case of a random effects model with binary data, which doesn't require external random covariates is the rather oddly termed *Negative Binomial regression*. Here the expected proportions π are assumed to have their own Gamma distribution. Another model is one where the random effect is Normally distributed. These models will be described in Chapter 5. When the variance is less than expected, it is known as "under-dispersion". This can happen if, for example, the data are being tampered with. Humans often underestimate the extent of random variation, so invented data tends to vary too little. Random effects models cannot deal with this since the model requires the random effect to increase the variance, but it may be possible to use generalised estimating equations (see Chapter 5) to deal with under-dispersion, since they don't require this property.

3.3.3 The Logistic Transform is Inappropriate

The logistic transform is not the only one that converts a probability ranging from 0 to 1 to a variable that, potentially, can range from minus infinity to plus infinity. Other examples are the *probit* transformation given by $probit(\pi) = \phi^{-1}(\pi)$ and the *complementary log-log* transform given by $\log[-\log(1-\pi)]$. The function ϕ is the cumulative Normal distribution (i.e. $\phi(x)$ that is the probability that a standard Normally distributed variable is less than x, so for example $\phi(0) = 0.5$) and ϕ^{-1} is the inverse so that $\phi(\text{probit}(\pi)) = \pi$). Probits are closely linked to logits and since the latter give odds they are generally preferred. The complementary log-log transform is useful when the events (such as deaths) occur during a cohort study and leads to survival analyses (see Chapter 4). Some packages enable one to use different link functions to see if one is better than the others. Usually they will give similar results.

3.4 Uses of Logistic Regression

1) As a substitute for multiple regression when the outcome variable is binary in cross-sectional and cohort studies and in clinical trials. Thus, we would use logistic regression to investigate the relationship between a causal variable and a binary output variable, allowing for confounding variables which can be categorical or continuous.

2) As a discriminant analysis to try and find factors that discriminate two groups. Here, the outcome would be a binary variable indicating membership to a group. For example, one might want to discriminate men and women on psychological test results.
3) To develop prognostic indicators, such as the risk of complications from surgery.
4) To develop diagnostic tools.
5) To analyse case-control studies and matched case-control studies.

3.5 Interpreting a Computer Output

Most computer packages have different procedures for the situations when the data appear in a grouped table and when they refer to individuals. It is usually easier to store data on an individual basis since it can be used for a variety of purposes. The coefficients and SEs of a logistic regression analysis will be exactly the same for the grouped procedure when the independent variables are all categorical and where the dependent variable is the number of successes in the group, and for the ungrouped procedure where the dependent variable is simply 0/1. In general, it is easier to examine the goodness-of-fit of the model in the grouped case.

3.5.1 One Binary Independent Variable

Consider the example given in *Statistics at Square One* of a trial of Isoniazid for the treatment of tuberculosis in children with HIV.

We can define an event as a child dying and we have a single categorical variable X_1 which takes the value 1 if the child is in the Isoniazid arm and 0 if they were in the placebo arm. The data are given in Table 3.2.

Table 3.2 Results for the Isoniazid trial after six months of follow-up.

	Dead	Alive	Total
Placebo	21	110	131
Isoniazid	11	121	132

We can rewrite Table 3.2 for the computer either as for a grouped analysis:

y (dead)	*n (total)*	Treatment (1 Isoniazid, 0 placebo)
21	131	0
11	132	1

or as the following 263 rows for an ungrouped analysis:

Row number	y Outcome		Treatment
	1 Dead, 0 Alive		(1 = Isoniazid, 0 = placebo)
1	1	(21 times)	0
22	0	(110 times)	0
132	1	(11 times)	1
143	0	(121 times)	1

One might use a grouped analysis if one did not have access to the raw data, but usually in a paper when there are several categorical covariates, tables comprise 2 × 2 tables of the outcome variable against each of the covariates separately. For example, the outcome variable may be cross-classified by gender and race separately but one could not then estimate the effect of race, *allowing* for gender. If a covariate is continuous, one could use group means as the covariate but it is usually better to keep the covariate as continuous and use an ungrouped analysis.

As described in *Statistics at Square One* the RR of death on Isoniazid relative to placebo is (11/132)/(21/131) = 0.52. The OR is (11/121)/(21/110) = 0.48. The reason for the discrepancy is that when the outcome, in this case death, is quite common the RRs and ORs tend to differ. When the outcome is rare (e.g. probability of an event < 0.1) then the OR and RR will be closer. In Chapter 6, we will show how to obtain the RR directly using regression. The usual analysis for a 2 × 2 table is the chi-squared test and in *Statistics at Square One* we get $X^2 = 3.645$, d.f. = 1, p = 0.056.

The model for these data is given in Equation 3.5 where π_i is the probability that individual i dies and $X_i = 0$ if individual *i* is in the Placebo group and $X_i = 1$ if individual i is in the Isoniazid group:

$$log_e\left(\frac{\pi_i}{1-\pi_i}\right) = log_e(o_i) = \beta_0 + \beta_1 X_i \tag{3.5}$$

When $X_i = 0$ Equation 3.5 becomes (1) $\log_e(O_0) = \beta_0$, and when $X_i = 1$ Equation 3.5 becomes (2) $\log_e(O_1) = \beta_0 + \beta_1$. Subtracting (1) from (2) we get $log_e\left(\frac{O_1}{O_0}\right) = \beta_1$, that is, the coefficient associated with treatment is the log OR of treatment compared to placebo.

A selection of the output from an R program for a logistic regression for the grouped data is shown in Table 3.3. The R code to produce this output is given in Appendix 5.

In Table 3.3, for the grouped data there are only two deviance residuals for the null model since there are only two groups. Their computation is given in Appendix A2. The deviance residuals for the fitted model are zero. The intercept is the estimate of β_0, which is the estimate of the log odds of dying in the Placebo group, so exp (−1.656) = 21/110 = 0.19. The Pr(>|z|) is the p-value and for the intercept is ridiculous since it is not testing a sensible hypothesis. The log OR for treatment is −0.7419. The two-sided p-value associated with this is derived from the z-value, assuming Normality (in R *2*pnorm(−1.879) = 0.0602*). This is

Table 3.3 Output from R logistic regression programs for grouped data from Table 3.2.

```
Grouped data
# Null model
Deviance residuals:
      1        2
  1.298   -1.419
# Fitted model
Deviance residuals:
[1]   0  0

Coefficients:
             Estimate Std. Error  z value  Pr(>|z|)
(Intercept)   -1.6560     0.2381   -6.954  3.56e-12
Treatment1    -0.7419     0.3948   -1.879    0.0602

(Dispersion parameter for binomial family taken to be 1)

Null deviance: 3.6982e+00 on 1 degrees of freedom
Residual deviance:  1.5543e-15 on 0 degrees of freedom

# log-likelihood
'log Lik.' -4.439942 (df=2)

AIC: 12.88
# Odds Ratio and 95% Confidence Interval

       OR        2.5 %    97.5 %
0.4761905   0.2196386 1.0324115
```

the Wald test, described in Appendix A2. A separate piece of code gives us the OR exp(−0.7419) = 0.48 with associated 95% CI. Note how the CI is asymmetric about 0.48, but just includes unity, as expected, since the p-value is greater than 0.05. R also states rather enigmatically that the: "dispersion parameter for binomial family taken to be 1." This means that the SEs are calculated assuming no over-dispersion as discussed in Section 3.3.2. Ways of checking this are described in the next paragraphs.

The Null deviance of 3.6982 is distributed as a chi-squared distribution with 1 degree of freedom and has associated probability *1-pchisq(3.6982, 1)* = 0.0544. This is the Likelihood Ratio test described in Appendix 2. The residual deviance is in fact zero because there are two groups and the model has two parameters. The AIC referred to in the output is the Akaike Information Criteria. It is based on the log likelihood but adds a penalty factor for the number of parameters included in the model.

$$\text{AIC} = 2\text{k} - 2\log(\text{likelihood})$$

In this case we get: $\text{AIC} = 2 \times 2 + 2 \times 4.44 = 12.88$

As we have just shown, if one had as many parameters as there were data points, one could fit the data exactly. The value of the AIC itself is not meaningful, but if you have a number of candidate models, the better model in general will be one with a smaller AIC.

The output for the ungrouped data is shown in Table 3.4.

Table 3.4 Output from R logistic regression programs for ungrouped data from Table 3.2.

```
Ungrouped data

# Null model
Deviance residuals:
    Min        1Q    Median       3Q       Max
-0.5094   -0.5094   -0.5094  -0.5094    2.0525

# Fitted model
Deviance residuals:
    Min        1Q    Median       3Q       Max
-0.5911   -0.5911   -0.4172  -0.4172    2.2293

Coefficients:
             Estimate Std. Error z value Pr(>|z|)
(Intercept)   -1.6560     0.2381  -6.954 3.56e-12
Treatment1    -0.7419     0.3948  -1.879   0.0602 .

(Dispersion parameter for binomial family taken to be 1)

    Null deviance: 194.75 on 262 degrees of freedom
Residual deviance: 191.05 on 261 degrees of freedom

# Log-likelihood

'log Lik.' -95.52539 (df=2)

AIC: 195.05
```

There are now as many deviance residuals as there are units, but as shown in Appendix A2 for the null model they only take two values and for the fitted model they take four values, corresponding to the entries in Table 3.2. The coefficients and SEs are exactly the same as for the grouped data, but here the residual deviance is not zero. The difference in the two deviances $194.75 - 191.05 = 3.70$ is distributed as a chi-squared with $262 - 261 = 1$ degree of freedom. The AIC is now $2 \times 2 + 2 \times 95.53 = 195.06$.

When the model comprises a single parameter, the three tests, the score test (the conventional chi-squared test), the Wald Test and the Likelihood Ratio test all test the same hypothesis. These three tests are compared in Table 3.5.

One can see that in this case the p-values are close together, with the Wald test giving a slightly larger p-value than the other two. It can be shown the Wald test is slightly less efficient (tends to give a slightly larger p-value) than the other two. As the sample size gets larger the three p-values will converge. As we shall see later, when the model comprises more than one parameter, the score test and the likelihood ratio test usually assess the model as a whole, whereas usually the Wald test tests each parameter,

Table 3.5 The three different p-values for a 2 × 2 table.

Test	P-value
Pearson X^2 test (score test)	0.056
Likelihood Ratio test	0.054
Wald test	0.060

although this doesn't have to be the case and we could use a likelihood ratio test to test each parameter.

3.5.2 Two Binary Independent Variables

Consider the data supplied by Julious and Mullee[5] on mortality of diabetics in a cohort study given in Table 3.6.

Table 3.6 Data from Julious and Mullee[5] on mortality of diabetics.

		Died	Total	%
Age < 40	Non-insulin dependent	0	15	0
	Insulin dependent	1	130	0.1
Age ≥ 40	Non-insulin dependent	218	529	41.2
	Insulin dependent	104	228	45.6
All ages	Non-insulin dependent	218	544	40.1
	Insulin dependent	105	358	29.3

Data from [5].

Note that over all ages a greater percentage of deaths occur in the non-insulin group, but when we split by age a greater proportion of deaths occurs in each of the insulin-dependent groups. This is an example of *Simpson's Paradox*. The explanation is that age is a confounding factor, since non-insulin-dependent diabetes is predominantly a disease of older age and, of course, old people are more likely to die than young people. In this case the confounding is so strong it reverses the apparent association.

The model we need to fit is:

$$log_e\left(\frac{\pi_i}{1-\pi_i}\right) = \beta_0 + \beta_1 X_{i1} + \beta_2 X_{i2} \tag{3.6}$$

where $X_{i1} = 1$ if subject i is insulin dependent and 0 otherwise and $X_{i2} = 1$ if subject i is aged ≥ 40 and 0 if aged < 40.

To analyse Table 3.6 we code the data for a grouped analysis as follows:

Dead	Total	Group	Age
		Dependent = 1 Non-dependent = 0	< 40 is 0 ≥ 40 is 1
0	15	0	0
1	130	1	0
218	529	0	1
104	228	1	1

Table 3.7 Selected output from R programs fitting logistic regression to data in Table 3.6.

```
# Model with the Insulin_Dependent as a covariate

                          OR      2.5%     97.5%     Pr(>|z|)
Insulin_Dependent 0.6206259 0.4667613 0.8252108 1.032284e-03

# Model with Insulin_Dependent and Age as covariates

                          OR        2.5%       97.5%     Pr(>|z|)
Insulin_Dependent    1.19919   0.8773042    1.639176 2.546655e-01
Age                118.88127  16.3954129  861.994489 2.277583e-06
```

The output from two logistic regressions with insulin dependent alone and then age and insulin dependent using data in Table 3.6 is given in Table 3.7.

In the first part of the analysis the OR associated with the group is 0.62, suggesting that insulin dependence has a lower risk of death than non-dependence. When age is included as a factor, this changes to an OR of 1.199. This estimate is basically a weighted estimate of the OR for people aged < 40 and the OR for those ≥ 40. It is greater than one and suggests an adverse effect of insulin dependence albeit non-statistically significant ($P = 0.255$). It should be stressed that this does not prove that starting to take insulin for diabetes *causes* a higher mortality; other confounding factors, as yet unmeasured, may also be important. Note the p-value for age is 2.28×10^{-6}. It should never be reported like this, since it cannot be justified to such extremely small values, but rather reported as $P < 0.001$, which is the smallest p-value worth quoting.

This procedure is the logistic equivalence to ANCOVA described in Section 2.5.1. Here the covariate, age, is binary, but it could be included as a continuous covariate and Julious and Mullee[5] show that including age as a continuous variable changes the RR to 1.15, which is similar to the ORs observed here.

As usual, one has to be aware of assumptions. The main one here is that the OR for insulin dependence is the same in the younger and older groups. There are not enough data to test that here. Another assumption is that the cut-off point at age 40 years was chosen on clinical grounds and not by looking at the data to file the best possible result for the investigator. One would need some reassurance of this in the text.

3.5.3 Two Continuous Independent Variables

A consecutive series of 170 patients were scored for risk of complications following abdominal operations with an APACHE risk score (a scoring system based on clinical signs and symptoms), which in this study ranged from 0 to 27 (Johnson *et al.*[6]). Their weight (in kg) was also measured. The outcome was whether the complications after the operation were mild or severe. Here both input variables are continuous. The output is given in Table 3.8 The interpretation of the model is that, *for a fixed weight*, a subject who scores one unit higher on the APACHE will have an increased OR of severe complications of 1.9 and this is highly significant ($P < 0.001$). Also note that a 1 kg increase in weight is associated with a 4% increase in the risk of complications.

The deviance residuals do not give any cause for concern. The minimum and maximum are plausible since one would expect values of roughly this size in 169 independent Normally distributed observations. It is important to check the overall significance of the model and this can be done by comparing the change in deviance when the parameters are

Table 3.8 Selection of R code to fit logistic regression to abdominal data (Johnson *et al.*[6]).

```
Deviance residuals:
     Min        1Q  Median      3Q      Max
 -2.3510   -0.4662 -0.1278  0.3743   2.4150

Coefficients:
             Estimate  Std. Error z value  Pr(>|z|)
(Intercept)  -8.83907    1.65729  -5.333  9.64e-08
apache        0.64105    0.10578   6.060  1.36e-09
weight        0.03879    0.01431   2.711   0.00671
---

(Dispersion parameter for binomial family taken to be 1)

    Null deviance: 220.74 on 169 degrees of freedom
Residual deviance:  113.73 on 167 degrees of freedom
AIC: 119.73

# Odds ratios and 95% confidence intervals
            OR      2.5 %     97.5 %
apache 1.898479  1.542993  2.335865
weight 1.039551  1.010803  1.069117

# Calculate LR chi2
[1] 107.0112

# Calculate Prob > chi2
[1] 5.791743e-24

# Calculate Hosmer-Lemeshow
     Hosmer and Lemeshow goodness of fit (GOF) test

X-squared = 4.9406, df = 8, p-value = 0.7639
```

added to the model. The change in deviance is 107 and under the null hypothesis that neither covariate is a predictor has a chi-squared distribution with 2 d.f. It can be seen from the output that this is very highly significant ($P = 5.29 \times 10^{-24}$).

The Hosmer–Lemeshow statistic (discussed in Section 3.3.1) is not statistically significant, indicating that the observed counts and those predicted by the model are quite close, and thus the model describes the data reasonably well. In practice, investigators use the Hosmer–Lemeshow statistic to reassure themselves that the model describes the data and so they can interpret the coefficients. However, one can object to the idea of using a significance test to determine goodness-of-fit, before using another test to determine whether coefficients are significant. If the first test is not significant, it does not tell us that the model is true, but only that we do not have enough evidence to reject it. Since no model is exactly true, with enough data the goodness-of-fit test will always reject the model. However, the model may be "good enough" for a valid analysis. If the model does not fit, is it valid to make inferences from the model? In general, the answer is "yes", but care is needed.

Other investigations might be to examine the sensitivity and specificity of the linear combination of APACHE score and weight to decide on an optimum cut-off for prediction. A further check on the model is to look at the influential points and see if there are a few that are critical to the results. These are now available in many statistical packages.

3.6 Examples in the Medical Literature

Stead *et al.*[7] wished to examine the views of people in England, Scotland and Wales on Covid-19 vaccination in January and February 2021. They conducted a nationally representative survey of 5931 adults and obtained responses for 4979. The main question is whether participants had had a Covid-19 vaccine or would accept a Covid-19 vaccine. The authors examined eight covariates to see which factors might affect acceptance. These were: gender (3 groups), age (7 groups), education status (5 groups), financial status (5 groups), country (England, Wales, Scotland), urban/rural, ethnicity (6 groups), Covid-19 status (6 groups), that is, 37 groups in total. Overall, the acceptance level was 83% (4137 out of 4979) who stated they had accepted/intended to accept the vaccine.

The results for ethnicity are show in Table 3.9.

Table 3.9 reproduces part of the results table given by Stead.[7] The third column shows the percentages who would accept the vaccine, weighted to allow for the fact that groups with different demographics have different response rates (e.g. older people are more likely to respond to a questionnaire and so would be overrepresented in a survey). The OR in column 4 (not given by the authors) is based on the weighted response rates, but not adjusted by logistic regression. Thus for "Any other white background" the OR is derived from the given data as: $0.46 = 0.758 \times (1 - 0.871)/\{0.871 \times (1 - 0.758)\}$.

The logistic regression analysis was based on the observed data, not on the weighted data, since all the characteristics believed to affect response rates were included in the model. The baseline for ethnicity was chosen as the largest group, White British. The interpretation of the Adjusted OR for "Any other white background" is that the odds of a person in this category accepting a vaccine are only 55% of those of white British person, of the same age, gender, educational status, etc. It is important to stress that because the actual proportions are large this is *not* the RR.

Table 3.9 Percentage of people accepting Covid-19 vaccine by ethnic group (extract of results table from Stead *et al.*[7]).

Ethnicity	N	% accepted[1]	OR[2]	AOR[3]	95% CI	P-value
White British	4226	87.1	1	1		
Any other white background	318	75.8	0.46	0.55	0.40 to 0.76	< 0.001
Mixed or multiple ethnic groups	82	61.4	0.24	0.39	0.21 to 0.71	< 0.001
Asian or Asian British	161	61.4	0.24	0.41	0.28 to 0.61	< 0.001
Black or black British	67	58.4	0.21	0.25	0.14 to 0.43	< 0.001
Other	50	72.8	0.40	0.42	0.23 to 0.79	0.007

(1) Weighted by population characteristics, (2) calculated from columns 2 and 3, (3) Adjusted Odds Ratio (AOR) for all covariates listed in previous paragraph.
Hosmer and Lemeshow: $X^2 = 7.44$, d.f. = 8, p = 0.49, final model: 1 $X^2 = 497$, d.f. = 29, p < 0.001.
Adapted from [7].

From some simple algebra it can be shown that from Equations 3.1 and 3.2 we can derive the RR from the OR:

$$RR = \frac{OR}{ORp_0 + 1 - p_0}$$

If there were only one binary covariate the variable, p_0 is the proportion of events in the reference category. A problem with multiple covariates is to know which value of p_0 to use to estimate the RR, since it will depend on a mixture of the covariates, but if we use the weighted White British proportion of 0.871 we find the RR for "any other white background": RR = 0.55/ (0.55 × 0.871 + 1 − 0.871) = 0.90. One can see that using the RR, which is more intuitive than the OR, changes the interpretation somewhat, in that a reduction of only 10% in the risk is not the impression conveyed by the OR of 0.55. It should be pointed out that this is *not* a good way to estimate the RR. A better way will be described in Chapter 5 under Poisson regression.

3.6.1 Comment

A key assumption of the model is that there are no interactions. For example, the AOR of 0.55 for Other white background relative to White British applies even overall. For example, people from the Other white background with a degree have an adjusted OR 0.55 of accepting the vaccine relative to White British with a degree. The authors do not say whether they checked for interactions. However, they do show the Hosmer–Lemeshow statistic, which is not significant. This suggests that all the covariates used give a reasonable description of the data and that adding other covariates, or interactions of the given covariates is unlikely to improve the fit by much. It is important to check that the overall model is significant, along with the individual parameters, since it is possible to find some parameters are statistically significant even if the overall model is not. In this case the overall model is statistically significant (p < 0.001). Note, one can derive the degrees of freedom of 29 by adding the number of groups from each covariate and subtracting the total number of covariates

(37 – 8). An issue here is called the "sparse data bias".[8] When the data are all categorical, it is possible that for some combinations of covariates there are few events, even for large data sets. Estimates of the OR for some combination of covariates may be severely biased. This will mean that the overall estimate of the OR is also biased. One simple check is to carry out some cross-tabulations to see if events are rare for some tables. A related issue is if the covariate predicts the outcome perfectly. If *b* and *c* in Equation 3.2 are 0, then the covariate predicts the outcome perfectly, but the OR is not defineable.[9] Most logistic regression programs struggle here. The reader is referred to Greenland *et al*[8] and Mansournia *et al*[9] for more sophisticated methods of dealing with this problem.

3.7 Case-control Studies

One of the main uses of logistic regression is in the analysis of case-control studies. It is a happy fact that an OR is reversible.[1] Thus, in Table 3.2 the OR is the same whether we consider the odds of a child dying on the Isoniazid arm, or the odds of being on the Isoniazid arm given that a child died. This reversal of logic occurs in case-control studies, where we select cases with a disease and controls without the disease. We then investigate the amount of exposure to a suspected cause that each has had. This is in contrast to a cohort study, where we consider those exposed or not exposed to a suspected cause, and then follow them up for disease development.

If we employ logistic regression, and code the dependent variable as 1 if the subject is a case and 0 if it is a control, then the estimates of the coefficients associated with exposure are the log ORs, which, provided the disease is relatively rare, will provide valid estimates of the RR for the exposure variable.

3.8 Interpreting Computer Output: Unmatched Case-control Study

Consider the meta-analysis of four case-control studies described in Altman *et al.*[10] from Wald *et al.* (Table 3.10).[11]

Table 3.10 Exposure to passive smoking among female lung cancer cases and controls in four studies.[11]

Study	Lung cancer cases		Controls		OR
	Exposed	Unexposed	Exposed	Unexposed	
1	14	8	61	72	2.07
2	33	8	164	32	0.80
3	13	11	15	10	0.79
4	91	43	254	148	1.23

Data from [11].

For the computer Table 3.10 is rewritten as:

Y (cases)	*n* (cases controls)	Exposed	Study
14	75	1	1
8	80	0	1
33	197	1	2
etc.			

In rewritten computer table there are eight rows, this being the number of unique study multiplied by the number of exposure combinations. The dependent variable for the model is the number of cases. One also has to specify the total number of cases and controls for each row. The output from a logistic regression program is given in Table 3.11. Here the *study* is a four-level categorical variable, which is a confounder and modelled with three dummy variables as described earlier in this chapter and in Chapter 2. This is known as a *fixed-effects* analysis. Chapter 5 gives a further discussion on the use of dummy variables where we might consider the effects as random. The baseline is arbitrarily chosen as Study 1, but the ORs given are not of interest, the dummies are there simply to control for the study effect so that we can get the exposure effect averaged over studies. The main result is that lung cancer and passive smoking are associated with an OR of 1.198, with 95% CI 0.858 to 1.672, which is not significant (p = 0.29).

Table 3.11 Output from a logistic regression program for the case–control study in Table 3.10.

```
Coefficients:
             Estimate Std. Error z value   Pr(>|z|)
(Intercept)  -1.8894     0.2465  -7.665   1.78e-14
Study2        0.1736     0.2928   0.593    0.55327
Study3        1.7455     0.3674   4.752   2.02e-06
Study4        0.6729     0.2522   2.668    0.00764
Exposed1      0.1803     0.1704   1.058    0.29001

    Null deviance: 32.8238  on 7  degrees of freedom
Residual deviance:  2.6726  on 3  degrees of freedom

AIC: 48.368

# Odds ratios and 95% confidence intervals
               OR      2.5 %     97.5 %
Study2    1.189557 0.6701409  2.111565
Study3    5.728823 2.7885268 11.769444
Study4    1.959967 1.1954634  3.213372
Exposed1 1.197527 0.8575806  1.672228
```

3.9 Matched Case-control Studies

In matched case-control studies each case is matched directly with one or more controls. For a valid analysis the matching should be taken into account. An obvious method would be to fit dummy variables as strata for each of the matched groups. However, it can be shown that this will produce biased estimates.[12] Instead we use a method known as *conditional logistic regression*. In a simple 2 × 2 table this gives a result equivalent to a McNemar's test.[1] It is a flexible method that with most modern software allow cases to have differing numbers of controls; it is not required to have exact 1:1 matching.

The logic for a *conditional* likelihood is quite complex, but the argument can be simplified. Suppose in a matched case-control study with exactly one control per case we had a logistic model such as Equation 3.3; for pair *i* the probability of an event for the control was π_{io} and for the case π_{i1}. Given that we know that one of the pair *must* be the case, that is, there must be one and only one event in the pair, *conditional* on the pair, the probability of the event happening for the case is simply $\omega_i = \pi_{i1} / (\pi_{io} + \pi_{i1}) = o_i/(1 + o_i)$, where $o_i = \pi_{i1} / \pi_{i0}$. As an example, suppose we knew that a husband and wife team had won the lottery; the husband had bought five tickets and the wife one, so he would be five times more likely to win than his wife given that other factors are the same, $o_i = 5$ and $\omega_i = 5/6$. Thus, the probability that the husband had won the lottery (knowing that either he or his wife had won) is a conditional probability of 5/6. We can form a conditional likelihood by multiplying the probabilities for each case-control pair ω_i, and maximise it in a manner similar to that for ordinary logistic regression and now this is simply achieved with many computer packages.

The model is the same as Equation 3.3, but the method of estimating the parameters is different, using conditional likelihood rather than unconditional likelihood. Any factor which is the same in the case-control set, for example a matching factor, cannot appear as an independent variable in the model.[1]

3.10 Interpreting Computer Output: Matched Case-control Study

These data are taken from Eason *et al.*[13] and described in Altman *et al.*[10] Thirty-five patients who died in hospital from asthma were individually matched for sex and age with 35 control subjects who had been discharged from the same hospital in the preceding year. The adequacy of monitoring of the patients was independently assessed and the results are given in Table 3.12.

For a computer analysis this may be written as a data-file with 35 × 2 = 70 rows, one for each case and control as shown in Table 3.13. For example, the first block refers to the ten deaths and ten survivors for whom monitoring is inadequate.

The logic for conditional logistic regression is the same as for McNemar's test. When the monitoring is the same for both case and control, the pair do not contribute to the estimate of the OR. It is only when they differ that we can calculate an OR.

From Table 3.14, the estimated OR of dying in hospital associated with inadequate monitoring is given by the ratio of the numbers of the two discordant pairs, namely 13/3 = 4.33.

The results of the conditional logistic regression are given in Table 3.14. The *p*-value for the Wald test is 0.022, which is significant, suggesting that inadequate monitoring increases

Table 3.12 Adequacy of monitoring in hospital of 35 deaths and 35 matched survivors with asthma.[13]

		Deaths (cases)	
		Monitoring	
		Inadequate	Adequate
Survivors	Inadequate	10	3
(Controls)	Adequate	13	9

Adapted from [13].

Table 3.13 Data from Table 3.12 written for a computer analysis using conditional logistic regression.

Pair number	Case–control (1 death 0 = survival)		Monitoring (1 = inadequate, 0 = adequate)
1	1		1
1	0		1
		(for 10 pairs)	
11	1		1
11	0		0
		(for 13 pairs)	
24	1		0
24	0		1
		(for 3 pairs)	
27	1		0
27	0		0
		(for 9 pairs)	

the risk of death. The *p*-value for the likelihood ratio (LR) test is 0.0094. Note the disparity between the LR test and the Wald test *p*-values. This is because the numbers in the table are small and the distribution discrete and so the approximations that all the methods use are less accurate. The McNemar's chi-square (a score test) is $(13 - 3)^2/(13 + 3) = 6.25$ with $P = 0.012$, which is mid-way between the LR and the Wald test. Each value can be regarded as valid, and in cases of differences it is important to state which test was used for obtaining the *p*-value. This is in contrast to linear regression in Chapter 2, where the three methods will all coincide.

The OR is estimated as 4.33 with 95% CI 1.23 to 15.21. This CI differs somewhat from the CI given in Altman *et al.*[10] because an exact method was used there, which is preferable with small numbers.

Table 3.14 Output from conditional logistic regression of the matched case-control study in Table 3.12.

```
             Coef exp(coef) se(coef)  z        p
Monitoring   1.47      4.33    0.641  2.29     0.022
Likelihood ratio test=6.74  on 1 df, p=0.00944, n=32

# OR
                    OR       2.5%     97.5%
Monitoring  4.333333  1.234857 15.20644
```

Note that the advantage of conditional logistic regression over a simple McNemar's test is that other covariates could be easily incorporated into the model. In the above example, we might also have measured the use of bronchodilators for all 70 subjects, as a risk factor for dying in hospital.

3.11 Example of Conditional Logistic Regression in the Medical Literature

Hojlund *et al.*[14] conducted a matched case control study to examine the association between the use of second generation antipsychotics (SGA) and the risk of incident chronic kidney disease (CKD) between 2001 and 2016 in Funen, Denmark. They found 21,434 cases with CKD and matched each by age, sex and calendar year of diagnosis to four controls from the general population who had had creatinine measured as normal and so were assumed not to have kidney disease. They used conditional logistic regression to analyse the data and gave the crude OR and the OR adjusted for prior use of lithium, recent use of NSAIDs, diabetes, hypertension and highest achieved level of education. In the cases they found 20,877 had never used SGAs whereas 557 had, and in the controls 83,845 had never used SGAs compared with 1731 who had. From this one can find a crude OR of 1.29.They found that ever users of SGA were at an increased risk of CKD, with an adjusted OR = 1.24, (95% CI 1.12 to 1.37).

3.11.1 Comment

The reason for matching is that it is assumed that CKD incidence relates to age, sex and year of diagnosis. Because the data are individually matched, conditional logistic regression should be used. The crude OR was not defined but coincided with the OR from the data, not allowing for matching. It can be seen that the crude OR and the adjusted OR are very close, suggesting the matching was not critical and so an ordinary logistic regression would give similar answers. The authors did some sensitivity analysis, in particular they looked at a dose-response relationship (number of prescriptions) and failed to find one. They suggest that SGAs do not directly increase the risk of CKD, but rather contribute to metabolic disturbances which result in kidney damage.

3.12 Alternatives to Logistic Regression

In recent years, computer intensive methods such as machine learning have been developed which ostensibly do the same job as logistic regression. We would argue that one needs a good grounding in logistic regression before one can understand machine learning. In addition, machine learning is good at making predictions, but does not explain how these predictions come about. We discuss this further in Section 1.11. There are numerous papers comparing the two, and for a recent review we suggest Levy and O'Malley.[15]

3.13 Reporting the Results of Logistic Regression

- Summarise the logistic regression to include the number of observations in the analysis, the coefficient of the explanatory variable with its SE and/or the OR and the 95% CI for the OR and the *p*-value.
- If a predictor variable is continuous then it is often helpful to scale it to ease interpretation. For example, it is easier to think of the increased risk of death every ten years than the increased risk per year, since the latter will be much closer to 1.
- Specify which type of *p*-value is quoted (e.g. LR or Wald test).
- Confirm that the assumptions for the logistic regression were met, in particular that the events are independent and the relationship plausibly log-linear. If the design is a matched one, ensure that the analysis uses an appropriate method such as conditional logistic regression.
- Report any sensitivity analysis carried out.
- Name the statistical package used in the analysis. This is important because different packages sometimes have different definitions of common terms.
- Specify whether the explanatory variables were tested for interaction.
- Report the underlying risks so some assessment can be made of the absolute risks involved.

3.14 Reading about the Results of Logistic Regression

In addition to the points in Sections 1.11 and 2.10.

- Is logistic regression appropriate? Is the outcome a simple binary variable? If there is a time attached to the outcome then survival analysis might be better (Chapter 4).
- The outcome is often described as "RRs". While this is often approximately true, they are better described as "approximate RRs", or better "ORs". Note that for an OR, a non-significant result is associated with a 95% CI that includes 1 (not 0 as in multiple regression).
- Has a continuous variable been divided into two to create a binary variable for the analysis? How was the splitting point chosen? If it was chosen after the data had been collected be very suspicious.

- Have any sensitivity tests been carried out? Is there evidence of over-dispersion?
- If the design is a matched case-control study, has conditional logistic regression been carried out?

3.15 Frequently Asked Questions

1) *Does it matter how the dependent variable is coded?*
   This depends on the computer package. Some packages will assume that any positive number is an event and 0 is a non-event. Changing the code from 0/1 to 1/0 will simply change the sign of the coefficient in the regression model.
2) *How is the OR associated with a continuous variable interpreted?*
   The OR associated with a continuous variable is the ratio of odds of an event in two subjects, in which one subject is one unit higher than another. This assumes a linear model which can be hard to validate. One suggestion is to divide the data into five approximately equal groups, ordered on the continuous variable. Fit a model with four dummy variables corresponding to the four higher groups, with the lowest fifth as baseline. Look at the coefficients in the model (not the ORs). If they are plausibly-increasing linearly, then a linear model may be reasonable. Otherwise, report the results of the model using the dummy variables.

3.16 Exercise

Stead[7] gave the following result for gender as shown in Table 3.15.

1) Find the crude OR for acceptance rates for males versus females and contrast with the adjusted OR.
2) Find the RR of acceptance for males versus females.
3) Are females statistically significantly less likely to accept the vaccine than males?
4) What does the overall chi-squared statistic tell us and why does it have two degrees of freedom?

Table 3.15 Vaccine acceptance by gender.

Gender	N	Vaccine acceptance	Adjusted OR	95% CI lower	95% CI upper
Male	2136	2097	1		
Female	2830	2788	0.82	0.67	0.99
Other	10	9	0.47	0.09	2.45

Adapted from [7].

$X^2\,(2) = 2.154$ $P = 0.341$

References

1 Beaumont R. *Health Science Statistics Using R and R Commander*. Banbury: Scion, 2015.

2 Hilbe J M. *Practical Guide to Logistic Regression*. Boca Raton, Florida: CRC Press, 2016.

3 Hosmer J D W, Lemeshow S, Sturdivant R X. *Applied Logistic Regression*. Chichester: John Wiley & Sons, 2013.

4 Feng C, Li L, Sadeghpour A. A comparison of residual diagnosis tools for diagnosing regression models for count data. *BMC Med Res Methodol* 2020; **20**(1): 1–21.

5 Julious S A, Mullee M A. Confounding and Simpson's Paradox. *Br Med J* 1994; **309**: 1480–1.

6 Johnson C D, Toh S K, Campbell M J. Combination of APACHE-II score and an obesity score (APACHE-O) for the prediction of severe acute pancreatitis. *Pancreatology* 2004; **4**: 1–6.

7 Stead M, Jessop C, Angus K, Bedford H, *et al.* National survey of attitudes towards and intentions to vaccinate against COVID-19: implications for communications. *BMJ Open* 2021; **11**(10): e055085. doi: 10.1136/bmjopen-2021-055085

8 Greenland S, Mansournia M A, Altman D G. Sparse data bias: a problem hiding in plain sight. *BMJ* 2016; **352**: i1981 doi:10.1136/bmj.i1981

9 Mansournia M A, Geroldinger A, Greenland S, Heinze G. Separation in logistic regression: causes, consequences, and control. *Am J Epidemiol* 2018; **187**(4): 864–70.

10 Altman D G, Machin D, Bryant T N, Gardner M J, eds. *Statistics with Confidence*. London: BMJ Books, 2000.

11 Wald N J, Nanchahal K, Thompson S G, Cuckle H S. Does breathing other people's tobacco smoke cause lung cancer? *Br Med J* 1986; **293**: 1217–22.

12 Breslow N E, Day N E. *Statistical Methods in Cancer Research 1: The Analysis of Case Control Studies*. Lyon: IARC, 1980.

13 Eason J, Markowe H L J. Controlled investigation of deaths from asthma in hospitals in the North East Thames region. *Br Med J* 1987; **294**: 1255–8.

14 Højlund M, Lund L C, Herping J L E, Haastrup M B, Damkier P, Henriksen D P. Second-generation antipsychotics and the risk of chronic kidney disease: a population-based case-control study. *BMJ Open* 2020; **10**(8): e038247.

15 Levy J J, O'Malley A J. Don't dismiss logistic regression: the case for sensible extraction of interactions in the era of machine learning. *BMC Med Res Methodol* 2020; **20**(1): 1–15.

References

[illegible]

4

Survival Analysis

Summary

When the dependent variable is a survival time, we need to allow for censored observations. We can display the data using a Kaplan–Meier plot. A useful model for modelling survival times on explanatory variables is known as a *proportional hazards* model, which is also referred to as a *Cox model*. It is a generalisation of the log-rank test, which is used for one binary independent variable, to allow for multiple independent variables that can be binary, categorical and continuous. It does not require a specification of an underlying survival distribution. A useful extension is to allow for stratification of an important categorical prognostic factor, so that subjects in different strata can have different underlying survival distributions.

4.1 Introduction

In survival analysis, the key variable is the time until some event. Commonly, it is the time from treatment for a disease to death, but, in fact, it can be time to any event. Examples include time for a fracture to heal and time that a nitroglycerine patch stays in place. As for binary outcomes, we imagine individuals having an event, but attached to this *event* is a *survival time*.

There are two main distinguishing features about survival analysis:

1) The presence of *censored observations*. These can arise in two ways. First, individuals can be removed from the data set without having an event. For example, in a study looking at survival from some disease, they may be lost to follow-up or get run over by a bus and so all we know is that they survived up to a particular point in time. Second, the study might be closed at a particular time point, as for example when a clinical trial is halted. Those still in the study are also regarded as censored, since they were alive when data collection was stopped. Clinical trials often recruit over a period of time, hence subjects recruited more recently will have less time to have an event than subjects recruited early on.

Statistics at Square Two: Understanding Modern Statistical Application in Medicine, Third Edition.
Michael J. Campbell and Richard M. Jacques.

2) The development of models that do not require a particular distribution for the survival times, the so-called *semi-parametric models*. This methodology allows a great deal of flexibility, with fewer assumptions than are required for fully parametric models.

A critical assumption in these models is that the probability that an individual is censored is unrelated to the probability that the individual has an event. If individuals who respond poorly to a treatment are removed before death and treated as censored observations, then the models that follow are invalid. This is the so-called *uninformative* or *non-informative censoring* assumption.

The important benefit of survival analysis over logistic regression, say, is that the time an individual spent in the study can be used in the analysis, even if they did not have an event. In survival, the fact that one individual spent only ten days in the study, whereas another spent ten years is taken into account. In contrast, in a simple chi-squared test or in logistic regression, all that is analysed is whether the individual has an event or not.

Further details are given in Collett,[1] and Machin *et al.*[2] Simple approaches to survival analysis have been given in *Statistics at Square One* and displaying survival data is described by Freeman *et al.*[3]

4.2 The Model

The dependent variable in survival analysis is what is known as the *hazard*. This is a probability of dying at a point in time, but it is conditional on surviving up to that point in time, which is why it is given a specific name.

Suppose we followed a cohort of 1000 people from birth to death. Say, for the age group 45–54 years, there were 19 deaths. In a 10-year age group there are 10 × 1000 *person-years at risk*. We could think of the death rate per person-year for 45–54-year-olds as 19/(10 × 1000) = 1.9 per 1000. However, if there were only 910 people alive by the time they reached 45 years of age, then the risk of death per person-year in the next 10 years, having survived to 45 years, is 19/(10 × 910) = 2.1 per 1000 per year. This is commonly called the *force of mortality*. In general, suppose X people were alive at the start of a year in a particular age group, and x people died during a period of width, t. The risk over that period is $x/(tX)$. If we imagine the width t of the interval getting narrower, then the number of deaths x will also fall but the ratio x/t will stay constant. This gives us the *instantaneous death rate* or the *hazard rate* at a particular time. (An analogy might be measuring the speed of a car by measuring the time t it takes to cover a distance x from a particular point. By reducing x and t, we get the instantaneous speed at a particular point.)

The model links the hazard to an individual i at time t, $h_i(t)$ to a baseline hazard $h_0(t)$ by:

$$log_e\left[h_i(t)\right] = log_e\left[h_0(t)\right] + \beta_1 X_{i1} + \ldots + \beta_p X_{ip} \tag{4.1}$$

where $X_{i1}, X_{i2} \ldots, X_{ip}$ are covariates associated with individual i.
This can also be written as:

$$h_i(t) = h_0(t)\exp(\beta_1 X_{i1} + \ldots + \beta_p X_{ip}) \tag{4.2}$$

The baseline hazard $h_0(t)$ serves as a reference point, and can be thought of as an intercept β_0 in multiple regression Equation 2.1. The important difference here is that it changes with time, whereas the intercept in multiple regression is constant. Similar to the intercept term, the hazard $h_0(t)$ in Equation 4.1 represents the death rate for an individual whose covariates are all 0, which may be misleading if, say, age is a covariate. However, it is not important that these values are realistic, but that they act as a reference for the individuals in the study.

Model 4.1 can be contrasted with model 3.3, which used the logit transform, rather than the log. Unlike model 3.3, which yielded odds ratios (ORs), this model yields *relative risks* (RR). Thus, if we had one binary covariate X, then $\exp(\beta)$ is the RR of (say) death for $X = 1$ compared to $X = 0$. Model 4.1 is used in *prospective* studies, where the RR can be measured.

This model was introduced by Cox[4] and is frequently referred to as the Cox regression model. It is called the proportional hazards model, because if we imagine two individuals, i and j, then 4.1 assumes that $h_i(t)/h_j(t)$ is constant over time; that is, even though $h_0(t)$ may vary, the two hazards for individuals whose covariates do not change with time remain proportional to each other. Since we do not have to specify $h_0(t)$, which is the equivalent of specifying a distribution for an error term, we have specified a model in 4.1 which contains parameters, and the model is sometimes described oxymoronically as *semi-parametric*. In the absence of censored observations (i.e. everyone has an event) the p-value for a Cox model with just a binary independent variable is close to that of the Mann-Whitney U test (*Statistics at Square One* Chapter 9) in the same way that linear regression with one binary independent variable gives a similar p-value to the t-test.

Given a prospective study such as a clinical trial, imagine we chose at random an individual *who has had an event* and their survival time is T. For any time t the survival curve $S(t)$ is $P(T \geq t)$, that is the probability of a random individual surviving longer than t. If we assume there are no censored observations, then the estimate of $S(t)$ is just the proportion of subjects who survive longer than t. When some of the observations can be censored it is estimated by the *Kaplan–Meier* survival curve described in *Statistics at Square One*. For any particular time t the hazard is:

$$h(t) = \frac{P(T = t)}{P(T \geq t)}$$

Suppose $S_0(t)$ is the baseline survival curve corresponding to a hazard $h_0(t)$ and $S_x(t)$ is the survival curve corresponding to an individual with covariates $X_{i1},\ldots, X_{ip}$. Then it can be shown that under model 4.1:

$$S_x(t) = S_0(t)\exp(\beta_1 X_{i1} + \ldots + \beta_p X_{ip}) \tag{4.3}$$

The relationship in Equation 4.3 is useful for checking the proportional hazards assumption, which we will show later.

The two important summary statistics are the number of events and the *person-years at risk*. There can only be one event per individual.

If more than 50% of events have occurred then from the Kaplan–Meier curve we can measure the median survival time, t_m, as the point when $S(t) = 0.5$. A simple model for survival is the exponential one where $S(t) = 1-\exp(-\lambda t)$. In this model the hazard λ is constant over time, Thus, a median survival time is given by is $0.5 = 1-\exp(-\lambda t_m)$ and so $\exp(-\lambda t_m) = 0.5$. Given a simple trial with treatment and controls hazards λ_1 and λ_0 respectively and median survival times t_1 and t_0 we have $\lambda_0 t_0 = \lambda_1 t_1$ and so $\lambda_0/\lambda_1 = t_1/t_0$. Thus, a simple interpretation of a hazards ratio, if we can assume the hazards remain constant, is simply the inverse ratio of the median survival. This may aid communication of a hazard ratio, roughly if a treatment has a hazard ratio for survival of 0.5 compared to control, that means the median survival time for people on treatment is doubled. An empirical investigation by Cortés *et al.*[5] has shown that this relationship holds approximately true on average over a large number of studies but with a high degree of uncertainty .

4.3 Uses of Cox Regression

1) As a substitute for logistic regression when the dependent variable is a binary event, but where there is also information on the length of time to the event. The time may be censored if the event does not occur.
2) To develop prognostic indicators for survival after operations, survival from disease or time to other events, such as time to heal a fracture.

4.4 Interpreting a Computer Output

The method of fitting model 4.1 is again a form of maximum likelihood, known as the *partial likelihood*. In this case, the method is quite similar to the matched case-control approach described in Chapter 3. Thus, one can consider any time at which an event has occurred, one individual (the case) has died and the remaining survivors are the controls. From model 4.1 one can write the probability that this particular individual is a case, given his/her covariates, compared to all the other survivors, and we attempt to find the coefficients that maximise this probability for all the cases. Once again computer output consists of the likelihood, the regression coefficients and their standard errors (SEs). *Statistics at Square One* describes the data given by McIllmurray and Turkie[6] on the survival of 49 patients with Dukes' C colorectal cancer. The data are given in Table 4.1.

It is important to appreciate that these are times from randomisation or entry to the study. The first person in the table may have only entered the study one month before the investigator decided to stop the trial. The subjects with large censored survivals might have

Table 4.1 Survival in 49 patients with Dukes' C colorectal cancer randomly assigned to either linolenic acid or control treatment (times with "+" are censored).

Treatment	Survival time (months)
γ-linolenic acid (n = 25)	1+, 5+, 6, 6, 9+, 10, 10, 10+, 12, 12, 12, 12, 12+, 13+, 15+, 16+, 20+, 24, 24+, 27+, 32, 34+, 36+, 36+, 44+
Control (n = 24)	3+, 6, 6, 6, 6, 8, 8, 12, 12, 12+, 15+, 16+, 18+, 18+, 20, 22+, 24, 28+, 28+, 28+, 30, 30+, 33+, 42

entered the study early, and have not had an event yet. In the computer, we have an "event" variable which takes the value 0 for a censored observation and 1 for an "event".

The data are entered in the computer as:

Time	Event	Group (1 = γ-linolenic acid, 0 = control)
1	0	1
5	0	1
6	1	1
etc.		

The Kaplan–Meier survival curve is shown in Figure 4.1. Note the numbers at risk are shown on the graph. The output for the Cox regression is shown in Table 4.2.

Ties in the data occur when two survival times are equal. There are a number of ways of dealing with these. The most common is known as *Breslow's method*, and this is an approximate method that will work well when there are not too many ties. Some packages will also allow an "exact" method, but this usually takes more computer time. An "exact" partial likelihood is shown here, because the large number of ties in the data may render approximate methods less accurately.

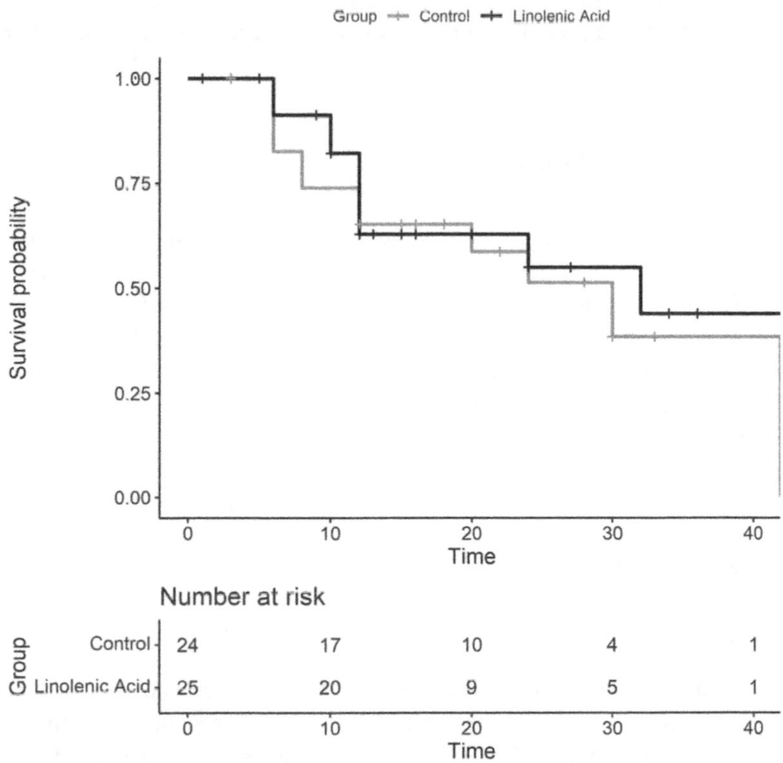

Figure 4.1 Kaplan–Meier survival plots for data in Table 4.1.

Table 4.2 Analysis of γ-linolenic acid data.

```
n= 49, number of events= 22
The coefficients
          coef  exp(coef)  se(coef)       z  Pr(>|z|)
Group -0.2755     0.7592     0.4488  -0.614     0.539

The Relative Risk
        exp(coef)  exp(-coef)  lower .95   upper .95
Group     0.7592        1.317      0.315        1.83

Concordance= 0.527 (se = 0.062)
Likelihood ratio test = 0.38 on 1 df, p=0.5
Wald test             = 0.38 on 1 df, p=0.5
Score (logrank) test  = 0.38 on 1 df, p=0.5

'log Lik.' -55.70416 (df=1)
```

From the output one can see that the hazard ratio associated with active treatment is 0.759 (95% CI 0.315 to 1.830). This has associated p-values of 0.5 by the likelihood ratio (LR), Wald and score (log-rank) methods, which implies that there is little evidence of efficacy. The risk and confidence interval (CI) are very similar to those given in *Statistics at Square One*, which used the log-rank test. An important point to note is that the z-statistic is *not* the ratio of the hazard ratio to its SE, but rather the ratio of the *regression coefficient* (log(hazard ratio)) to *its* SE.

4.5 Interpretation of the Model

In model 4.1, the predictor variables can be continuous or discrete. If there is just one binary predictor variable X, then the interpretation is closely related to the log-rank test.[4] In this case, if the coefficient associated with X is b, then $\exp(b)$ is the *relative hazard* (often called the relative risk (RR)) for individuals for whom $X = 1$ compared with $X = 0$. When there is more than one covariate, then the interpretations are very similar to those described in Chapter 3 for binary outcomes. In particular, since the linear predictor is related to the outcome by an exponential transform, what is additive in the linear predictor becomes multiplicative in the outcome, as in logistic regression Section 3.1.

4.6 Generalisations of the Model

4.6.1 Stratified Models

Suppose we had two groups and we did not wish to assume that the incidence rate for one group was a constant multiple of the incidence rate of the other. For example we might have severe disease (SD) and mild disease (MD). It may seem unreasonable to expect SD to be constant risk over time relative to MD. Then we can fit two separate models to the two groups:

1) for the SD:

$$log_e\left[h_{iSD}(t)\right] = log_e\left[h_{0SD}(t)\right] + \beta_1 X_{i1} + \ldots + \beta_p X_{ip}$$

2) and for the MD:

$$log_e\left[h_{iMD}(t)\right] = log_e\left[h_{0MD}(t)\right] + \beta_1 X_{i1} + \ldots + \beta_p X_{ip}$$

This is known as a *stratified Cox model*. Note that the regression coefficients, the βs – for the covariates other than the stratifying one are assumed to remain constant. Say X_1 was a binary variable, gender, where 1 is if the person is female. Then the baseline, males, will have different risks depending on whether they are in the severe or mild disease groups, and females will also have different risks for severe and mild disease. However, the ratio of male to female risks will be the same in the severe and mild disease. This is an extension of the idea of fitting different intercepts for a categorical variable in multiple regression.

The analysis is still a conditional one; here we are conditioning on separate strata. This is similar to the analysis of matched case-control studies where the matching is on the case-control group. The important point is that the stratum effect is removed by conditioning; one does not have to use a fixed or random effects model to model it.

4.6.2 Time Dependent Covariates

The model 4.1 assumes that the covariates are measured once at the beginning of the study. However, the model can be generalised to allow covariates to be time dependent. An example might be survival of a cohort of subjects exposed to asbestos, where a subject changes jobs over time and therefore changes his/her exposure to the dust. These are relatively easily incorporated into the computer analysis.

4.6.3 Parametric Survival Models

Another generalisation is to specify a distribution for $h_0(t)$ and use a fully parametric model. A common distribution is the *Weibull distribution*, in which $S(t) = 1-\exp(-(t\lambda)^{\beta})$ is a generalisation of the exponential distribution and becomes the exponential distribution when $\beta = 1$. This leads to what is known as an *accelerated failure time model*, and this is so-called because the effect of a covariate X is to change the time scale by a factor exp($-\beta$). Thus rather than, say, a subject dies earlier, one may think of them as simply living faster. Details of this technique are beyond the scope of this book, but it is widely available on computer packages. Usually it will give similar answers to the Cox regression model. It is useful when one wants to estimate an *average* survival required, for example in health economics, rather than a *median*, which can be obtained from the Kaplan–Meier plot.

4.6.4 Competing Risks

A further generalisation occurs when we might have two kinds of outcome, for example deaths due to cancer and deaths due to other causes. If we can assume that deaths due to other causes is completely independent of deaths due to cancer then we could treat deaths due to other causes as censored. If not, then we have what are called *competing risks.* Dealing with these properly is beyond the scope of this book, but a safe approach would be to simply treat, for example, all deaths as events rather than looking at different causes (a dead person does not care about what caused the death).

4.7 Model Checking

The assumption about linearity of the model is similar to that in multiple regression modelling described in Section 2.6 and can be checked in the same way. The methods for determining leverage and influence are also similar to those in multiple regression and hence we refer the reader to Section 2.7. There are a number of ways of calculating residuals, and various packages may produce some or all of *martingale residuals, Schoenfeld residuals* or *deviance residuals*. Details are beyond the scope of this book. However, since the Cox model is semi-parametric, the exact distribution of the residuals is unimportant.

The new important assumption is that the hazard ratio remains constant over time. This is most straightforward when we have two groups to compare with no covariates. The simplest check is to plot the Kaplan–Meier survival curves for each group together. If they cross, then the proportional hazards assumption may be violated. For small data sets, where there may be a great deal of error attached to the survival curve, it is possible for curves to cross, even under the proportional hazards assumption. However, it should be clear that an overall test of whether one group has better survival than the other is meaningless, when the answer will depend on the time that the test is made. A more sophisticated check is based on what is known as the *complementary log-log plot*. Suppose we have two groups with survival curves $S_1(t)$ and $S_2(t)$. We assume that the two groups are similar in all prognostic variables, except group membership. From Equations 4.1 and 4.3, if the proportional hazard assumption holds true, then:

$$log_e\left\{-\log_e\left[S_1(t)\right]\right\} = k + log_e\left\{\log_e\left[S_2(t)\right]\right\}$$

where k is a constant. This implies that if we plot both: $log_e\left\{-log_e(S_1(t))\right\}$ and: $log_e\left\{-log_e(S_2(t))\right\}$ against either log(t) or t, then the two curves will be parallel, with distance k apart.

This graph is plotted for the data in Table 4.1, and shown in Figure 4.2. It can be seen that the two curves overlap considerably, but there is no apparent divergence between them and so they are plausibly parallel.

There are also a number of formal tests of proportional hazards and further details are given in Machin *et al.*[2] Most packages will provide a number of such tests. As an example, Table 4.3 shows the result of a test of proportional hazards, based on the Schoenfeld residuals. It can be seen that this agrees with the intuitive graphical test that there is little evidence of a lack of proportional hazards.

The problems of testing proportional hazards are much more difficult when there are a large number of covariates. In particular, it is assumed that the proportional hazards assumption remains true for one variable independent of all the other covariates. In practice, most of the covariates will simply be potential confounders, and it is questionable

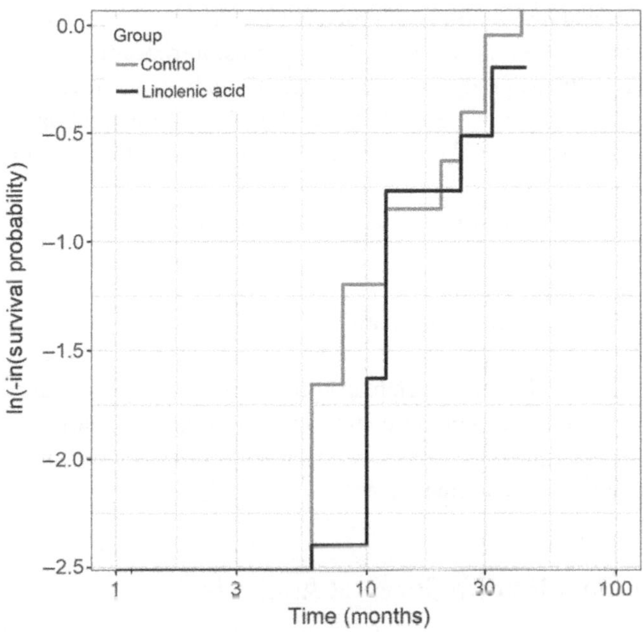

Figure 4.2 Log-log plot of survival curves in Figure 4.1.

Table 4.3 Test of proportional hazards assumption (computer output).

	chisq	df	p
GLOBAL	0.0128	1	0.91

whether statistical inference is advanced by assiduously testing each for proportionality in the model. It is important, however, that the main predictors, for example treatment group in a clinical trial, be tested for proportional hazards because it is impossible to interpret a fixed estimated RR if the true risk varies with time.

The other assumptions about the model are not testable from the data, but should be verified from the protocol. These include the fact that censoring is independent of an event happening. Thus, in a survival study, one should ensure that patients are not removed from the study just before they die. Survival studies often recruit patients over a long period of time and so it is also important to verify that other factors remain constant over the period, such as the way patients are recruited into a study and the diagnosis of the disease.

4.8 Reporting the Results of a Survival Analysis

Useful reviews on the reporting of survival analysis haves been given by Dey *et al.*[7] and Batson *et al.*[8]

- Specify the nature of the censoring, and as far as possible validate that the censoring is non-informative.
- Report the total number of events, subjects and person-time of follow-up, with some measure of variability, such as a range for the latter. For a trial this should be done by treatment group.

- Report an estimated survival rate at a given time, by group, with CIs.
- Display the Kaplan–Meier survival curves by group. To avoid misinterpretation of the right-hand end, terminate the curve when the number at risk is small, say 5. It is often useful to show the numbers at risk by group at regular time intervals, as shown in Figure 4.1. For large studies, this can be done at fixed time points, and shown just below the time axis.
- For smaller studies the censored observations could be marked on the Kaplan–Meir plots.
- Specify how median follow-up was calculated.
- Specify the regression model used; note sensitivity analyses undertaken and tests for proportionality of hazards.
- Specify a measure of risk for each explanatory variable, with a CI and a precise *p*-value. Note that these can be called RRs, but it is perhaps better to refer to relative hazards.
- Report the computer program used for the analysis. Many research articles just quote Cox[4] without much evidence of having read that paper.

4.9 Reading about the Results of a Survival Analysis

Is the proportional hazards assumption reasonable and has it been validated? A review of papers reporting survival analysis found that the majority who used Cox regression did not report any tests for proportional hazards or did not state criteria by which a graphical analysis could decide whether proportional hazards held true.[8]

- Has the modelling strategy been clearly described? For example, how did the authors decide which covariates to include in the model? Was this decided having analysed the data?
- Is there an overall fit to the model given?
- Are the conclusions critically dependent on the assumptions? For example, does it matter if proportional hazards are not quite true?
- Can we be sure that the censored observations are non-informative?
- In trials, are numbers of censored observations given by treatment group and in observational studies are they given by exposure group separately?
- Similar to the discussion in Chapter 3, what matters to patients is an absolute risk, not the RR. Are absolute risks given?

4.10 Example in the Medical Literature

In a cohort study, Nyberg *et al.*[9] examined the risk of hospital admission within 14 days after a positive Covid test for 839,278 patients, of whom 36,233 had been admitted to hospital in the UK between 23 November 2020 and 31 January 2021. They were interested in whether people having the B.1.1.7 variant (Alpha) of the virus were more at risk than people having earlier variants. They used S-gene target failure (SGTF) as a proxy for a person having the Alpha type variant.

The authors fitted two Cox models: a stratified one in which the baseline hazard is estimated separately for each set of confounder combinations, and one in which there was an assumed underlying hazard, and all the confounders (except age) were assumed to act multiplicatively of the baseline. In this model they also included exact age, IMD rank (a measure of multiple deprivation) and exact date within each of their respective categorical variables. They used this latter model to estimate absolute risks. The confounders they used were: ten year-age groups (nine groups), sex (two groups), ethnicity (six groups), index of multiple deprivation fifth (five groups), region of residence (nine groups), and week of specimen (ten groups). They used Schoenfeld tests to test for deviation from the proportional hazard assumption, and they visually assessed the assumption by examining log-log transformed Kaplan–Meier plots for SGTF status and each potential confounder.

Models including interactions between covariates and SGTF status indicated no effect modification except for age ($P < 0.001$), with little difference in hospital admission by SGTF status in patients under 20 but rising to hazard ratios in the range 1.45–1.65 in those aged 30 and older. The proportional hazards assumption was violated for other covariates for this model ($P < 0.001$). However, this may have reflected a high power to detect minor deviations from proportionality owing to the large sample size, and the corresponding log-log plots showed approximately parallel curves.

The authors concluded that results suggest that the risk of hospital admission is higher for people infected with the Alpha variant compared with earlier variants, likely reflecting a more severe disease. The higher severity may be specific to adults older than 30 years.

The results are shown in Table 4.4 for the overall model and for those aged 20–29 years.

4.10.1 Comment

This is an excellent paper because they describe the various tests they use to check the model. Good points are: (1) It is a large study so the results are reliable; (2) The authors found statistically significant departures from proportional hazards but decided from the log-log plots that these arose simply because of the high power due to large numbers and the departures were not great and did not influence the results; (3) The authors tested all the covariates for interaction with the main causal factor.

Table 4.4 Partial results of cohort study by Nyberg *et al.*[9]

SGTF status	No. (%) admitted to hospital	Stratified model Hazard Ratio 95%CI	Regression model Hazard Ratio 95% CI
All ages			
SGTF	27710/592,409 (4.7)	1.52 (1.47–1.57)	1.51 (1.47–1.55)
Non-SGTF	8523/246,869 (3.5)	1 (reference)	
20–29 years			
SGTF	2149/115,296 (1.9)	1.29 (1.16–1.43)	1.30 (1.19–1.42)
Non-SGTF	707/45,562 (1.6)	1 (reference)	

Data from [9].

Note that the week the specimen is taken is a time-dependent covariate. It is useful to include it because in a fast-moving epidemic the proportions infected with Alpha will increase rapidly over the follow-up period. One can also use it to check if its severity remains constant over the follow-up period, by looking at an interaction between SGTF status and the week thc specimen was taken.

In the first Cox model, because of the large number of strata, they found 22% of the individuals were in uninformative strata. Uninformative strata were defined as strata with zero hospitalisation events in at least one of the comparison groups (SGTF/non-SGTF) in the stratified model. Fitting the regression model avoids having to drop these subjects but highlights the possibility of the "sparse data problem" (Mansournia *et al.*[10]) whereby some subgroups might have extreme results. It is encouraging that the results are so similar for the stratified and regression model so this is unlikely to be serious.

Censoring, which is losing track of people before they are admitted to hospital was unlikely to be a problem. Only 911 (0.15%) patients with SGTF variants and 399 (0.16%) of those without SGTF variants died within 14 days without previous hospital admission; so how deaths were treated would make little difference to the hazard ratio estimates for hospital admission. It was assumed that if people were not on the lists of admissions to hospital within 14 days, then they were not admitted and not simply lost to follow-up. This begs the question as to whether a Cox model is needed. A logistic regression could have been done instead, since there were few censored observations before follow-up, but since the overall risk of admission was small, the ORs and hazard ratios would have been very similar. It is also good that one can compute the absolute risk difference (1.2% overall, 0.3% for those aged 20–29); the authors do not give a CI for the difference but rather for the absolute risks in each group. However, it is to be noted that the STROBE checklist does not require a risk difference, but a measure of absolute risk.[11] This is sensible since a model for a risk difference would be quite different to a model for the RR, and unlikely to describe the data well. For example it is more plausible that the RR is constant over strata which have different absolute risks, but this would mean that the absolute risk differences were not constant over strata and would require a more complex model.

4.11 Frequently Asked Questions

1) *Does it matter how the event variable is coded?*
   Unlike logistic regression, coding an event variable 1/0 instead of 0/1 has a major effect on the analysis. Thus, it is vitally important to distinguish between the events (say deaths) and the censored times (say survivors). This is because, unlike ORs, hazard ratios are not symmetric to the coding and it matters if we are interested in survival or death. For example, if in two groups the mortality was 10% and 15%, respectively, we would say that the second group has a 50% increased mortality. However, the survival rates in the two groups are 90% and 85%, respectively, and so the second group has a $5/90 = 6\%$ reduced survival rate.
2) *Does a test for proportional hazards matter if the test for group differences is not significant?*
   A statistical test of a group effect asks whether, over the whole time period, the hazards were greater in one group than another. However, if two survival curves cross, it

is easy to show that a treatment could have a worse survival early in the time period, but a beneficial effect later on, but overall there was no benefit. Thus it is important to actually look at the Kaplan–Meier and log-log plots to assist the interpretation of the survival curve.

4.12 Exercises

Exercise 4.1

Using the Results of Nyberg *et al.*[9] (Table 4.4)

a) Compute the number of strata in the stratified model.
b) Contrast the crude RR with the overall hazard ratio. Why is there a difference?
c) Is the hazard for people aged 20–29 statistically significantly different to the overall risk?
d) Is the proportional hazards assumption reasonable and has it been validated?
e) Is the conclusion that hospital admissions are higher in people affected by the Alpha variant critically dependent on the assumption of proportional hazards?
f) Are numbers of censored observations given by exposure group?
g) Is an absolute risk difference given?

Exercise 4.2

Campbell *et al.*[12] describe a cohort study over 24 years of 726 men exposed to slate dust and 529 controls. They used a Cox regression to examine the effect of slate dust exposure on mortality. They stratified by age group (ten years) in the analysis. They measured smoking habit and forced expiratory volume (FEV_1 a measure of lung function in litres) at baseline.

They found the following results:

		Hazard ratio	95% CI	*P*-value
Model 1	Slate	1.21	1.02–1.44	0.032
Model 2	Slate	1.24	1.04–1.47	0.015
	Smokers[a]	2.04	1.54–2.70	< 0.001
	Ex-smokers[a]	1.46	1.07–1.98	0.016
Model 3	Slate	1.17	0.97–1.41	0.11
	Smokers[a]	1.96	1.44–2.67	< 0.001
	Ex-smokers[a]	1.46	1.05–2.03	0.046
	FEV_1	0.74	0.65–0.83	< 0.001

[a] Relative to non-smokers.

a) Describe the findings. Include in your explanation the reason for using a stratified analysis.
b) Why do you think the hazard ratio for slate changes little when smoking habit is included in the model and yet becomes non-significant when FEV_1 is included.

c) State two major assumptions underlying model 2 and how they might be tested.
d) Interpret the coefficient for FEV_1 in model 3.

References

1 Collett D. *Modelling Survival Data in Medical Research*, 3rd edn. London: CRC Press, 2015.
2 Machin D, Cheung YB, Parmar M. *Survival Analysis: A Practical Approach*, 2nd edn. Chichester: John Wiley & Sons, 2006.
3 FreemanJV, WaltersSJ, CampbellMJ. *How to Display Data*. BMJ Books, Oxford: Blackwell Publishing, 2008.
4 Cox DR. Regression models and life tables (with discussion). *J Roy Statist Soc B* 1972; **34**: 187–20.
5 Cortés J, González JA, Campbell MJ, Cobo E. A hazard ratio can be estimated by a ratio of median survival times but with considerable uncertainty. *J Clin Epidemiol* 2014; **67**: 1172–7.
6 McIllmurray MB, Turkie W. Controlled trial of γ-linolenic acid in Duke's C colorectal cancer. *BMJ* 1987; **294**: 1260. **295**: 475.
7 Dey T, Mukherjee A, Chakraborty S. A practical overview and reporting strategies for statistical analysis of survival studies. *Chest* 2020; **158**(1): S39–48.
8 Batson S, Greenall G, Hudson P. Review of the reporting of survival analyses within randomised controlled trials and the implications for meta-analysis. *PLoS ONE* 2016; **11**(5): e0154870.
9 Nyberg T, Twohig KA, Harris RJ, *et al.* Risk of hospital admission for patients with SARS-CoV-2 variant B. 1.1. 7: cohort analysis. *BMJ* 2021; **373**(1412): doi:10.1136/bmj.n1412
10 Mansournia MA, Geroldinger A, Greenland S, Heinze G. Separation in logistic regression: causes, consequences, and control. *Am J Epidemiol* 2018; **187**(4): 864–70.
11 STROBE Checklists – STROBE (strobe-statement.org)
12 Campbell MJ, Hodges NG, Thomas HF, Paul A, Williams JG. A 24-year cohort study of mortality in slate workers in North Wales. *J Occup Med* 2005; **55**: 448–53.

5

Random Effects Models

Summary

Random effects models are used when there is more than one source of random variation. They are useful in studies where the observations can be grouped; being within a particular group affects the observations in that group and so the observations within a group are not independent. The models are useful in the analysis of *repeated measures* studies, *cluster randomised trials*, *multi-centre trials* and in *meta-analysis*. Ignoring the correlation of observations within groups can lead to underestimation of the standard error (SE) of key estimates. There are two types of models: *cluster specific* and *marginal models*. Marginal models treat the intra-cluster correlation (ICC) as a nuisance and utilise a technique known as *generalised estimating equations* (*gee*). Cluster specific models have specific terms for the random effects and use some form of maximum likelihood to estimate the coefficients of the model.

5.1 Introduction

In the previous chapters there has been only one source of random variation. This is the sampling error for each individual. We sample n individuals from a population. How might the estimates of our model vary by sampling a different set of n individuals? As we showed earlier, one of the great things about statistical inference is that we can use the variation between individuals to enable us to make predictions as to how estimates would vary if we had taken a different sample. However, we could sample within samples to get so-called multistage sampling. It is convenient to start with to think about two-stage sampling. We sample groups and then look at individuals within those groups. We could sample surgeons and then look at a sample of their patients to look at survival rates from different operations. We could sample individuals and then follow them up over time. There are now two sources of variation: between groups and between individuals within those groups.

The models described so far only have one error term. In multiple regression, as described by model 2.1, the error term was an explicit variable, ε, added to the predictor. In logistic regression, the error was Binomial and described how the observed and predicted values were related. However, possibilities are there for more than one error term. A simple

Statistics at Square Two: Understanding Modern Statistical Application in Medicine, Third Edition.
Michael J. Campbell and Richard M. Jacques.

example of this is when observations are repeated over time on individuals. There is then the random variation *within individuals* (repeating an observation on an individual does not necessarily give the same answer) and random variation *between individuals* (one individual differs from another). Another example would be the one in which each doctor treats a number of patients. There is *within-doctor variation* (since patients vary) and *between-doctor variation* (since different doctors are likely to have different effects on their patients). These are often known as *hierarchical data structures* since there is a natural hierarchy, with one set of observations nested within another. One form of model used to fit data of this kind is known as a *random effects model*. This is a vast topic and this chapter can no more than alert the reader to its importance and recommend further reading.

5.2 Models for Random Effects

Consider a randomised trial, where there are single measurements on individuals, but the individuals form distinct groups, such as being treated by a particular doctor.

For continuous outcomes, y_{ij}, for an individual j in group i, we assume that:

$$y_{ij} = \beta_0 + z_i + \beta_1 X_{1ij} + \ldots + \beta_p X_{pij} + \varepsilon_{ij} \tag{5.1}$$

This model is very similar to Equation 2.1, with the addition of an extra term z_i.

Here z_i is assumed to be a random variable with: $E(z_i) = 0$ and $Var(z_i) = \sigma_B^2$. This reflects the overall effect of being in group i and the X_{pij} s are the covariates on the pth covariate on the jth individual in the ith group with regression coefficients β_p.

We assume, $Var(\varepsilon_{ij}) = \sigma^2$ that z_i and ε_{ij} are uncorrelated and so, $Var(y_{ij}) = \sigma^2 + \sigma_B^2$

Thus, the variability of an observation has two components: the within- and the between-group variances.

The observations within a group are correlated and:

$$Corr(y_{ij}, y_{ij'}) = \rho = \frac{\sigma_B^2}{\sigma^2 + \sigma_B^2} \text{ if } j \text{ and } j' \text{ differ.}$$

The parameter ρ is known as the *intra-cluster (group) correlation* (ICC).

It can be shown that when a model is fitted, which ignores the z_is, the SE of the estimate of β_i is usually too small, and thus in general is likely to increase the type I error rate. In particular, if all the groups are of the same size, m, then the variance of the estimate increases by $1 + (m-1)\rho$ and this is known as the *design effect* (*DE*).

For some methods of fitting the model, we also need to assume that z_i and ε_{ij} are Normally distributed, but this is not always the case.

Model 5.1 is often known as the *random intercepts model*, since the intercepts are $\beta_0 + z_i$ for different groups i and these vary randomly. They are a subgroup of what is known as *multi-level models*, since the different error terms can be thought of as being different levels of a hierarchy, individuals nested within groups. They are also called *mixed models* because they mix random effects and fixed effects. Model 5.1 is called an *exchangeable model* because it would not affect the estimation procedure if two observations within a cluster were exchanged. Another way of looking at exchangeability, is that from Equation 5.1, given a value for z_i, the correlation between y_{ij} and $y_{ij'}$ is the same for any individuals j and j' in the same group. (This is also sometimes called the *sphericity* assumption.) An alternative model for longitudinal data is that errors are related in some way to how closely they are measured in time. The usual assumption is that: $corr(\epsilon_{ij}, \varepsilon_{ij'}) = k\alpha^{|j-j'|}$ where $|k| \leq 1$ and $0 \leq \alpha \leq 1$ is the autocorrelation coefficient. This model assumes the correlation between two variables gets smaller when they are distant in time. This is discussed further in Chapter 8

Random effects models can be extended to the Binomial and Poisson models. As the random effect induces variability above that predicted by the model they are often called *over-dispersed* models. A common extension of the Poisson is the *Negative Binomial* (see Chapter 6 for a discussion of Poisson models). Survival models can also be extended to include random effects, in which case the random effect is commonly known as the *frailty*.

Further details of these models are given in Brown and Prescott.[1] Repeated measures are described in Crowder and Hand,[2] and Diggle *et al.*[3] and the hierarchical models are described by Goldstein.[4]

5.3 Random vs Fixed Effects

Suppose we wish to include a variable in a model that covers differing groups of individuals. It could be a generic description, such as "smokers" or "non-smokers", or it could be quite specific, such as patients treated by Doctor A or Doctor B. The conventional method of allowing for categorical variables is to fit dummy variables as described in Chapter 2. This is known as a *fixed effect model*, as the effect of being in a particular group is assumed fixed and represented by a fixed population parameter. Thus, "smoking" will decrease lung function by a certain amount on average. Being cared for by Doctor A may also affect your lung function, particularly if you are asthmatic. However, Doctor A's effect is of no interest to the world at large, in fact it is only so much extra noise in the study. However, the effect of smoking is of interest generally. The main difference between a fixed and a random effects model depends on the intention of the analysis. If the study were repeated, would the same groups be used again? If not, then a random effects model is appropriate. By fitting dummy variables we are removing the effect of the differing groups as confounders. However, if these groups are unique to this study, and in a new study there will be a different set of groups, then we are pretending accuracy that we do not have since the effects we have removed in the first study will be different in a second study. Thus, random effects are sources of "error" in a model due to individuals or groups over and above the unit "error" term and, in general, the SEs of the fixed components will be greater when a random component is added

5.4 Use of Random Effects Models

5.4.1 Cluster Randomised Trials

A cluster randomised trial is one in which groups of patients are randomised to an intervention or control rather than individual patients. The group may be a geographical area, a general or family practice or a school. A general practice trial actively involves general practitioners and their primary health care teams, and the unit of randomisation may be the practice or health care professional rather than the patient. The effectiveness of the intervention is assessed in terms of the outcome for the patient.

A model for a simple cluster trial is:

$$y_{ij} = \beta_0 + z_i + \beta_1 X_{1ij} + \beta_2 X_{2ij} + \varepsilon_{ij}$$

Here, y_{ij} is the outcome from the ith individual in the jth practice, $X_{1ij} = 1$ if the jth practice is in the treatment group and $X_{1j} = 0$ is in the control; X_2ij is some covariate attached to patient i, for example the baseline value of the outcome. The covariates can be cluster level (i.e. they don't vary within a cluster) such as practice characteristics or patient level covariates which do vary within a custer.

There are many different features associated with cluster randomised trials and some of the statistical aspects were first discussed by Cornfield.[5] They have been discussed extensively by Campbell and Walters.[6] The main feature is that patients treated by one health care professional tend to be more similar than those treated by different health care professionals. If we know which doctor a patient is being treated by we can predict slightly better than by chance the performance of the patient and thus the observations for one doctor are not completely independent. What is surprising is how even a small correlation can greatly affect the design and analysis of such studies. For example with an ICC of 0.05 (a value commonly found in general practice trials), and 20 patients per group, the usual SE estimate for a treatment effect, ignoring the effect of clustering, will be about 30% lower than a valid estimate should be. This greatly increases the chance of getting a significant result even when there is no real effect (a type I error).

Further discussion on the uses and problems of cluster randomised trials in general (family) practice has been given by Campbell.[7]

5.4.2 Repeated Measures

A repeated measures study is where the same variable is observed on more than one occasion on each individual. There may be confusion over the difference between *a repeated measures analysis, a longitudinal analysis* and a *time series analysis.*

Repeated measures are usually many series, from different individuals, and the purpose of repeating the observations may be to improve the accuracy of the estimate of some parameter. Often the order does not matter. Longitudinal data measures individuals (or groups) over time, but the order is important. A time series is usually a single series, such as daily deaths in a country, where the purpose is to monitor the series or make predictions about future observations. Time series analysis is discussed in Chapter 8.

Consider blood pressure monitoring. My doctor tells me to take my blood pressure in the morning and evening every day for a week. These data form a time series, but in fact all the doctor requires is the mean value over the week. The reason for repeating the measure is to try and reduce the variability of the mean. Any information in the ordering is lost in the mean. An example of longitudinal data might be a clinical trial of a treatment to reduce blood pressure, where the blood pressure is measured 3, 6, 12 and 24 weeks after treatment. If the primary endpoint had been blood pressure at 24 weeks then measurements at other times are only secondary (but often useful for imputing any missing values at 24 weeks). However, if the primary endpoint was simply to see if treatment reduced blood pressure then all measurements count equally. Using the data at each time point one can see the time trends, for example a linear trend downward from baseline, or a drop by three weeks and a flat response afterwards. It is a debatable point whether one can choose a time response curve to fit to the data *after* viewing the data.

A simple method of analysing data of this type is by means of summary measures.[8–10] Using this method we simply find a summary measure for each individual, often just the average of the observations over time, and analyse this as the primary outcome variable. This then eliminates the within-individual variability and therefore we have only one error term, due to between-individual variation, to consider. Other summary values might be the maximum value attained over the time period, the slope of the line or the area under the time curve (AUC).

However, data may not be collected for some individuals for some time points. Summary measures are taken over different numbers of points and so their variability is different and this is not allowed for in a summary measures analysis. Random effects models are a flexible method of dealing with this. Each individual will have an effect on blood pressure, measured by the variable z_i. The individuals themselves are a sample from a population, and the level of blood pressure of a particular individual is not of interest. The random effect induces a correlation between measures within an individual, measured by the ICC. However, *conditional* on the random effect the observations are uncorrelated. Random effects models are also useful when the data are repeated, but some data are missing (see Section 1.10 in Chapter 1).

Note that there are many methods described as *repeated measures analysis of variance* which also tackle the analysis of repeated measures but they are often restricted to Normally distributed continuous outcomes. It is our experience that either using a summary measures approach, or modelling the random effects directly are easier to understand and communicate.

A trial design that mixes clustering and repeated measures is a longitudinal *stepped-wedge design*.[11] In this design all subjects start on the control group and then at given periods of time a subset of clusters are randomised to the intervention until all subjects/clusters are on the intervention. It is beyond the scope of this book.

5.4.3 Sample Surveys

Another simple use of the models would be in a sample survey, for example to find out levels of depression in primary care. A random sample of practices is chosen and within them a random sample of patients. The effect of being cared for by a particular practice on an individual is not of prime interest. If we repeat the study we would have a different set of practices. However, the variation induced on the estimate of the proportion of depressed patients by different practices *is* of interest, as it will affect the confidence interval (CI). Thus, we need to allow for between-practice variation in our overall estimate.

5.4.4 Multi-centre Trials

Multi-centre trials enroll subjects from more than one site. They are useful for evaluating treatments of rare diseases and also ensure reproducibility of the treatment effect across a broad range of characteristics that distinguish the sites. A useful analogy would be that of an individual patient data meta-analysis (see Chapter 7), where each centre can be regarded as a separate study. The crucial difference here is not just whether the treatment effect can be assumed random, but whether the centre effect itself is random (i.e. the centre affects the outcome for both the intervention and thc control). Strictly speaking, centres should be considered a random effect only when they are selected randomly from a population of centres. In practice, of course, they are volunteers, with prior experience or a special interest in the disease or treatment. The use of random effects models here is somewhat controversial. If the number of centres is small (say < 10), then modelling centres as either fixed or random can produce conflicting results, and the random effects models are more conservative. It is wise to consult an experienced statistician on these issues.[12]

5.5 Ordinary Least Squares at the Group Level

Cornfield[5] stated that one should "analyse as you randomise". Since randomisation is at the level of the group, a simple analysis would be to calculate "summary measures", such as the mean value for each group, and analyse these as the primary outcome variable.

Omitting the covariates from the model for simplicity, except for a dummy variable δ_i which takes the value 1 for the intervention and 0 for the control, it can be shown that:

$$\overline{y}_i = \mu + \tau\delta_i + \overline{\epsilon_i} \tag{5.2}$$

where $\overline{y}_i$ is the mean value for the n_i individuals with outcome, y_{ij}, $j = 1,...,n_i$ for group i and:

$$Var(\overline{y}_i) = \sigma_B^2 + \frac{\sigma^2}{n_i} \tag{5.3}$$

Equation 5.2 is a simple model with independent errors, which are homogeneous if each n_i is of similar size. An OLS estimate at group level of τ is unbiased and the SE of estimate is valid provided the error term is independent of the treatment effect.

Thus, a simple analysis at the group level would be the following: if each n_i is the same, or not too different, carry out a two-sample *t*-test on the group level means. This is the method of summary measures mentioned in Section 5.4.2. It is worth noting that if σ^2 is 0 (all values from a group are the same) then group size does not matter. An alternative method of analysis is to carry out a weighted analysis using as weights the inverse of the variance in Equation 5.3. (Given data: $x_i\,(i=1,\ldots,n)$ and a set of weights w_i a weighted mean is given by: $\overline{x}_{weighted} = \sum_i w_i x_i / \sum_i w_i$). The terms σ_B^2 and σ^2 can be estimated using an analysis of variance. If σ_B^2 can be assumed 0 the weights are simply the inverse of the sample sizes. This is the *fixed effect* analysis.

There are a number of problems with a group-level approach. The main one is how should individual level covariates be allowed for? It is unsatisfactory to use group averaged values of the individual-level covariates. Also this method ignores the fact that the summary measures may be estimated with different precision for different individuals. The advantage of random effects models over summary measures is that they can allow for covariates which may vary with individuals. They also allow for different numbers of individuals per group.

5.6 Interpreting a Computer Output

5.6.1 Different Methods of Analysis

There are at least four valid methods of analysing random effects data and (at least) one invalid method. The invalid one is to ignore the clustering. The other four that we will discuss are: using summary measures; using robust standard errors; using generalized estimating equations; and using maximum likelihood. The robust standard error (SE) is a simple method to inflate the SE obtained from OLS to allow for the increased variance caused by the random effect, which is discussed in more detail in Appendix 3. We have already discussed the summary measure approach.

5.6.2 Likelihood and gee

Many computer packages will now fit random effects models, although different packages may use different methods of fitting model 5.1. Since ignoring the random effect means the standard errors of the parameters are underestimated, a simple approach is to use so-called robust standard errors (Appendix 3). There are a huge variety of these, being robust to different assumptions, and it is important to state which method is used. This may not be very efficient and the usual approach would be a likelihood method. This first assumes a distribution (usually Normal) for each z_i and then formulates a probability of observing each y_{ij} conditional on each z_i. Using the distribution of each z_i we can obtain an expected probability over every possible z_i. This involves mathematical integration and is difficult to do. Since the method calculates the regression coefficients separately for each group or cluster, this is often known as the *cluster specific model*. A simpler method is known as *generalised estimating equations* (*gee*) which does not require Normality of the random effects. This method essentially uses the mean values per group as the outcome, and adjusts the SE for the comparison to allow for within group correlation using the *cluster robust or sandwich estimator* described in Appendix 3. The gee methodology is based on what is known as a *marginal model*. In an ordinary cross-tabulation of data, the means are given on the edges or margins of the table; hence the name marginal model. As the group or cluster is the main item for analysis, gee methodology may be unreliable unless the number of clusters exceeds 20, and preferably 40.

The methods can be extended to allow for Binomial errors, so that one can get random effect logistic regression. This type of model is generalised quite naturally to a Bayesian approach (see Appendix 4). This is beyond the scope of this book, but further details are given in, for example, Turner *et al.*[13]

5.6.3 Interpreting Computer Output

Table 5.1 gives some data which are a subset of data from Kinmonth *et al.*[14] They consist of the BMI at one year after randomisation on a number of patients in ten practices, under one of two treatment groups.

Table 5.2(i) shows the results of fitting an ordinary regression without clustering, which yields an estimate of a treatment effect of 0.42, with SE 1.904. As was stated earlier, since this ignores the clustering inherent in the data, the SE will be too small. Table 5.2(ii) shows the results of fitting the model using robust standard errors. One can see that the estimate of the treatment effect is the same but the SE is estimated as 2.776, which is much greater than in model (i). The robust SE method allows for heterogeneity in the variances between and within subjects. It also effectively weights the cluster means with the sample size of the cluster, giving the same mean as the unweighted estimate. The maximum likelihood model weights the estimates depending on the within and between cluster variances and yields an estimate of the treatment effect of 0.3917, with SE 2.4677. This estimate will be different if (possibly by chance) the estimate of an effect is (say) larger for larger clusters. If there is no

Table 5.1 Data on BMI.[14]

Subject	BMI (kg/M^2)	Treat	Practice
1	26.2	1	1
2	27.1	1	1
3	25.0	1	2
4	28.3	1	2
5	30.5	1	3
6	28.8	1	4
7	31.0	1	4
8	32.1	1	4
9	28.2	1	5
10	30.9	1	5
11	37.0	0	6
12	38.1	0	6
13	22.1	0	7
14	23.0	0	7
15	23.2	0	8
16	25.7	0	8
17	27.8	0	9
18	28.0	0	9
19	28.0	0	10
20	31.0	0	10

Data from [17].

real association between size of effect and size of cluster, then for large samples the methods will give similar results. Usually it is reasonable to assume no association, but one might imagine that (say) a teaching method is more effective if a group is small and so small groups have larger effects. Note again how the SE is inflated compared to the model that fails to allow for clustering. The output also gives the between-groups variance (Practice, an estimate of our model σ_B^2) and within-groups (Residual, an estimate of our σ^2) variance. From this we can get the ICC as $13.97/(13.97 + 2.37) = 0.85$. As a default, R gives the profile based CIs rather than the Wald ones (Appendix 2) since these don't require the estimate to have a Normal distribution.

Using the method of gee, given in Table 5.2(iv), yields a treatment estimate of 0.3862, but an SE of 2.459. As described earlier, the assumption underlying the analyses in (ii), (iii) and (iv) is that individuals within a group are *exchangeable.*

The estimate from gee can be contrasted with the method which uses the average per group (a summary measure) as the outcome in Table 5.2(v). This yields an estimate of 0.407, with an even larger SE of 2.748. This method does not weight the cluster means differently, so a small cluster will contribute the same as a large cluster.

The methods will give increasingly different results as the variation between groups increases. In this example the estimate of the treatment effect is quite similar for each method, but the SEs vary somewhat. The choice of method will depend on factors such as the number of clusters and the size of each cluster. Any method which allows for clustering is acceptable. If the methods give markedly different results then this should be investigated. It can occur, for example, if there is a clear relation between effect size and cluster size.

Table 5.2 Computer output fitting regression models to data in Table 5.1.

(i) Regression not allowing for clustering.

```
Residuals:
   Min      1Q Median      3Q     Max
-6.290 -2.630 -0.450  2.115  9.710

Coefficients:
             Estimate Std.  Error t  value Pr(>|t|)
(Intercept)    28.390       1.347   21.083 3.87e-14
Treatment       0.420       1.904    0.221    0.828
---

Residual standard error: 4.258 on 18 degrees of freedom
Multiple R-squared:  0.002695,  Adjusted R-squared:  -0.05271
F-statistic: 0.04864 on 1 and 18 DF,  p-value: 0.8279

# Confidence intervals
                   2.5 %      97.5 %
(Intercept)    25.560906   31.219094
Treatment      -3.580944    4.420944
```

(Continued)

Table 5.2 (Continued)

(ii) Regression with robust SEs.

```
Standard error type:  CR2

Coefficients:
              Estimate Std. Error t value  Pr(>|t|) CI Lower CI Upper    DF
(Intercept)     28.39      2.598 10.9270 0.0003984   21.176   35.604 4.000
Treatment        0.42      2.776  0.1513 0.8836850   -6.047    6.887 7.551

Multiple R-squared:  0.002695,  Adjusted R-squared:  -0.05271
F-statistic: 0.0229 on 1 and 9 DF,  p-value: 0.8831
```

(iii) Maximum likelihood random effects model.

```
Random effects:
 Groups   Name        Variance Std.dev.
 Practice (Intercept)   13.97    3.737
 Residual                2.37    1.540
Number of obs: 20, groups:  Practice, 10

Fixed effects:
            Estimate Std. error      df t value Pr(>|t|)
(Intercept)  28.3900     1.7409  9.9823  16.308  1.6e-08
Treatment     0.3917     2.4677 10.0629   0.159    0.877
---

# Confidence intervals
                 2.5 %    97.5 %
(Intercept)  24.621900  32.158101
Treatment    -4.941644   5.733615
```

(iv) Generalised estimating equations.

```
 Coefficients:
            Estimate Std. err    Wald  Pr(>|W|)
(Intercept)  28.3900   2.3239 149.250    <2e-16
Treatment     0.3862   2.4590   0.025     0.875
---

Correlation structure = exchangeable
Estimated Scale Parameters:

            Estimate Std. err
(Intercept)    16.32      7.8
  Link = identity

Estimated correlation parameters:
      Estimate Std. err
alpha   0.7971   0.1099
Number of clusters:   10  maximum cluster size: 3

# Confidence intervals

            Estimate Std. err      Wald Pr(>|W|)   lower   upper
(Intercept)  28.3900    2.324 149.25006   0.0000  23.835  32.945
Treatment     0.3862    2.459   0.02467   0.8752  -4.433   5.206
```

Table 5.2 (Continued)

(v) Regression on group means.

```
Coefficients:
              Estimate Std. Error t value Pr(>|t|)
(Intercept)    28.390      1.943   14.61  4.7e-07
Treatment       0.407      2.748    0.15     0.89
---

Residual standard error: 4.35 on 8 degrees of freedom
Multiple R-squared:  0.00273,   Adjusted R-squared:  -0.122
F-statistic: 0.0219 on 1 and 8 DF,  p-value: 0.886

# Confidence intervals
             2.5  %  97.5 %
(Intercept)  23.909  32.871
Treatment    -5.931   6.744
```

5.7 Model Checking

Most of the assumptions for random effects models are similar to those of linear or logistic models described in Chapters 2 and 3. The main difference is in the assumptions underlying the random term. Proper checking is beyond the scope of this book, but the maximum likelihood method assumes that the random terms are distributed Normally. If the numbers of measurements per cluster are fairly uniform, then a simple check would be to examine the cluster means, in a histogram. This is difficult to interpret if the numbers per cluster vary a great deal. In cluster randomised trials, it would be useful to check that the numbers of patients per cluster is not affected by treatment. Sometimes, when the intervention is a training package, for example, the effect of training may be to increase recruitment to the trial, so leading to an imbalance in the treatment and control arms.

5.8 Reporting the Results of Random Effects Analysis

- Recall that measuring one person twice is not the same as measuring two people once. The degrees of freedom for the main analysis are determined by the number of independent units. For example in a repeated measures analysis where the main unit is people, one should not have the degrees of freedom exceeding the number of people.
- In a cluster randomised trial, give the number of *groups or clusters* as well as the number of individuals. In a repeated measures or longitudinal study, give the number of *observations* as well as the number of individuals.
- Give the ICC.
- In a cluster randomised trial, give the group level means of covariates by treatment arm, so the reader can see if the trial is balanced *at a group level.*
- Describe whether a cluster specific, a marginal model or a summary measure is being used and justify the choice.
- Indicate how the assumptions underlying the distribution of the random effects were verified.

- Cluster randomised trials and stepped wedge trials now have a CONSORT statement to help report these areas.[15,16]
- State the type of robust SE and the method of computing the CI (e.g. Wald or profile).

5.9 Reading about the Results of Random Effects Analysis

- What is the main unit of analysis? Does the statistical analysis reflect this? Repeating a measurement on one individual is not the same as making the second measurement on a different individual and the statistical analysis should be different in each situation.
- Does the study report the ICC?
- If the study is a cluster randomised trial, was an appropriate model used?
- If the analysis uses gee methodology, are there sufficient groups to justify the results?

5.10 Examples of Random Effects Models in the Medical Literature

5.10.1 Cluster Trials

The REPOSE cluster randomised controlled trial compared the effectiveness of insulin pumps with multiple daily injects for adults with type 1 diabetes.[17] Participants were allocated to a Dose Adjustment for Normal Eating (DAFNE) structured education training course and then courses were randomised in pairs to receive either DAFNE plus insulin pump (156 participants on 23 courses) or DAFNE plus multiple daily injections (161 participants on 23 courses). The primary outcome for the trial was change in HbA1c after two years in participants whose baseline HbA1c was ≥ 7.5%. Participants allocated to one DAFNE course will have more similar outcomes than participants allocated to a different DAFNE course, the primary outcome was therefore compared between the two treatment groups using a linear mixed model with DAFNE course as a random intercept and centre and baseline HbA1c as fixed effect covariates. After two years the mean difference in HbA1c change from baseline was –0.24% (95% CI: –0.53% to 0.05%) in favour of the insulin pump treatment. The observed intraclass correlation coefficient was approximately 0.5%.

Note that the individuals were not randomised individually; they were allocated a cluster and then that was randomised to a pumps course or multiple daily injection course. The reason for doing this is that the investigators wanted to get consent from participants to the *trial*, knowing they could get either. It was possible that participants might enter the trial so as to get a pump but withdraw if they were allocated injections and this design reduced this possibility. Thus the random effect was the cluster, since this would differ if the trial were to be repeated and the fixed effect is the different type of course. One might ask why centres were not treated as random as well. The design of the study meant that each centre would have an equal number of both types of course so the centre effect was removed from the treatment comparisons. It was included as a fixed effect to examine whether a centre effect remained.

5.10.2 Repeated Measures

Doull *et al.*[18] looked at the growth rate of 50 children with asthma before and after taking inhaled steroids. They showed that, compared to before treatment, the difference in growth rate between weeks 0 and 6 after treatment was –0.067 mm/week (95% CI –0.12 to –0.015), whereas at weeks 19–24, compared to before treatment, it was –0.002 (95% CI –0.054 to 0.051). This showed that the growth suppressive action of inhaled corticosteroids is relatively short-lived.

5.10.3 Comment

The random effects model enabled a random child effect to be included in the model. It allowed differing numbers of measurements per child to be accounted for. The model gives increased confidence that the results can be generalised beyond these particular children.

5.10.4 Clustering in a Cohort Study

Reijman *et al.*[19] describe a cohort study of 1904 men and women with arthritis followed up for 6 years aged 55 years and over. They defined progression of hip osteoarthritis as a joint space narrowing of 1.0 mm or a total-hip replacement. The unit of measurement was the person and the measurement of the hip was clustered within the person. There were 2918 hips.

They used logistic regression via gee equations to test for predictors and allow for correlation between hips. They selected variables to go in the multivariate analysis using a univariate p-value of 0.1 They found a Kellgren and Lawrence grade ≥ 2 to have an odds ratio of 5.8 (95% CI 4.0 to 8.4) and that 89.7% were correctly predicted by the model.

5.10.5 Comment

The use of gees allowed a mixture of people with both hips measured, or only one hip measured to be included in the analysis. They did not justify a 1 mm narrowing of joint space as the cut-off for progression, but the use of a dichotomy enabled hip replacements to be included as an outcome and also made the assessment of the predictive ability easy. Note that since the model was developed on the same data as the prediction, applying the model to new data would result in fewer correct predictions. The endpoint is "composite" which can lead to problems.[20] Use of univariate tests to include in a multivariate model is not recommended (Section 1.9). They did not report the ICC between hips within people.

5.11 Frequently Asked Questions

1) *How can I tell if an effect is random or not?*
   If one wishes to generalise a result, then the effect is fixed. For example, when one

studies treatments in clinical trials or exposures in epidemiological studies one wishes to infer some form of causality and these effects therefore need to be fixed.

2) *Given the plethora of methods that can be used to analyse random effects model, which should I use?*
   This will depend on a number of factors, such as availability of software and size of sample. One is warned not to use gee methods if the number of clusters is less than about 20. If the numbers of subjects per cluster is similar then all methods will produce similar results. A key question is whether the treatment effect varies with the cluster size. This could be investigated by trying several methods which weight the estimates differently and see if they give markedly different results. If they do differ, then the reasons should be investigated.

5.12 Exercises

Exercise 5.1

Given an individually randomised controlled trial of an inhaled steroid against placebo, where measurements are made weekly for six weeks, which are random and which are fixed effects and which form part of the random error?
a) patient, b) treatment c) age group d) smoking group e) height f) measurements within patients.

Exercise 5.2

Given a cluster randomised controlled trial of a new type of counselling for depression, in which counsellors are randomised to be trained in one of two different techniques and for which levels of depression are assessed after six months of therapy, which are random and which are fixed effects and which form part of the random error?
a) counsellors, b) type of therapy, c) level of depression initially, d) patients

Exercise 5.3

Part of the results in Reijman *et al.*[19] are given in Table 5.3.

Table 5.3 Outcome Joint space narrowing of 1.0 mm or more or a total-hip replacement with six years of follow-up.

Predictor	OR (95% CI)
Age (years)	**1.06 (1.04 to 1.08)**
Sex (female)	**1.8 (1.4 to 2.4)**

Data from [19].

a) What are the possible problems with the outcome measure? What are the advantages?
b) What are the assumptions about the model?
c) If one person was 55 years old and another 65 years old at baseline, what are the increased odds of progression in the 65-year-old relative to a 55-year-old? What about a 75-year-old compared to a 65-year-old?
d) If 13% of men had progression, what percentage of women will have progressed?

References

1 Brown H, Prescott R. *Applied Mixed Models in Medicine*, 3rd edn. Chichester: John Wiley, 2015.
2 Crowder M, Hand DJ. *Analysis of Repeated Measures*. London: Taylor and Francis ebook, 2020.
3 Diggle PJ, Heagerty P, Liang K-Y, Zeger S. *Analysis of Longitudinal Data*, 2nd edn. Oxford: Oxford Science Publications, 2002.
4 Goldstein H. *Multi-level Models*, 4th edn. Chichester: Wiley, 2011.
5 Cornfield J. Randomization by group: a formal analysis. *Am J Epidemiol* 1978; **108**: 100–102.
6 Campbell MJ, Walters SJ. *How to Design, Analyse and Report Cluster Randomised Trials in Medicine and Health Related Research*. Chichester: Wiley-Blackwell, 2014.
7 Campbell MJ Cluster randomised trials. *The Medical Journal of Australia* 2019; **210**(4): 154–56. doi: 10.5694/mja2.13001
8 Matthews JNS, Altman DG, Campbell MJ, Royston JR. Analysis of serial measurements in medical research. *BMJ* 1990; **300**: 230–35.
9 Frison L, Pocock SJ. Repeated measures in clinical trials: analysis using mean summary statistics and its implications for design. *Statistics in Medicine* 1992; **11**(13); 1685–704.
10 Walters SJ, Campbell MJ, Machin D. *Medical Statistics: A Commonsense Approach*, 5th edn. Chichester: John Wiley, 2019.
11 Campbell MJ, Hemming K, Taljaard M. The stepped wedge cluster randomised trial: what it is and when it should be used. *The Medical Journal of Australia* 2019; **210**(6): doi: 10.5694/mja2.50018
12 Senn S. Some controversies in planning and analyzing multi-center trials. *Stat Med* 1998; **17**: 1753–65.
13 Turner RM, Omar RZ, Thompson SG. Bayesian methods of analysis for cluster randomized trials with binary outcome data. *Stat Med* 2001; **20**(3): 453–72.
14 Kinmonth AL, Woodcock A, Griffin S, Spiegal N, Campbell MJ. Randomised controlled trial of patient centred care of diabetes in general practice: impact on current well-being and future disease risk. *BMJ* 1988; **317**: 1202–08.
15 Campbell MK, Piaggio G, Elbourne DR, Altman DG. Consort 2010 statement: extension to cluster randomised trials. *BMJ* 2012; **4**: 345.
16 Hemming K, Taljaard M, McKenzie JE, *et al.* Reporting of stepped wedge cluster randomised trials: extension of the CONSORT 2010 statement with explanation and elaboration. *BMJ* 2018; **363**: 1614.

17 The REPOSE Study Group. Relative effectiveness of insulin treatment over multiple daily injections and structured education during flexible intensive insulin treatment for type 1 diabetes: cluster randomised trial (REPOSE). *BMJ* 2017; **356**: j1285.

18 Doull IJM, Campbell MJ, Holgate ST. Duration of growth suppressive effects of regular inhaled corticosteroids. *Arch Dis Child* 1998; **78**: 172–73.

19 Reijman M, Hazes JM, Pols HA, *et al*. Role of radiography in predicting progression of osteoarthritis of the hip: prospective cohort study. *BMJ* 2005; **330**: 1183.

20 Brown PM, Rogne T, Solligård E. The promise and pitfalls of composite endpoints in sepsis and COVID-19 clinical trials. *Pharmaceutical Statistics* 2021; **20**: 413–17. doi: 10.1002/pst.2070

6

Poisson and Ordinal Regression

Summary

This chapter will consider two other regression models which are of considerable use in medical research: *Poisson regression and ordinal regression*. Poisson regression is useful when the outcome variable is a count. Ordinal regression is useful when the outcome is ordinal, or ordered categorical.

6.1 Poisson Regression

Poisson regression is an extension of logistic regression where the risk of an event to an individual is small, but there are a large number of individuals, so the number of events in a group is appreciable. We need to know not just whether an individual had an event, but for how long they were followed up, the *person-years*. This is sometimes known as the amount of time they were *at risk*. It is used extensively in epidemiology, particularly in the analysis of cohort studies. For further details see Clayton and Hills.[1]

6.2 The Poisson Model

The outcome for a Poisson model is a count of events in a group, usually over a period of time, for example number of deaths over 20 years in a group exposed to asbestos. It is a *discrete quantitative variable* in the terminology of Chapter 1. The principal covariate is a measure of the amount of time the group have been in the study. Subjects may have been in the study for differing length of times (known as the *at risk period*) and so we record the time each individual is observed to give an exposure time e_i. In logistic regression we modelled the probability of an event π_i. Here we model the underlying rate λ_i which is the number of events expected to occur over a period i, E_i, divided by the time e_i. Instead of a logistic transform we use a simple log transform.

Statistics at Square Two: Understanding Modern Statistical Application in Medicine, Third Edition.
Michael J. Campbell and Richard M. Jacques.

The model is:

$$log_e(\lambda_i) = log\left(\frac{E_i}{e_i}\right) = \beta_0 + \beta_1 X_{i1} + \ldots + \beta_p X_{ip} \quad (6.1)$$

This may be rewritten as:

$$E_i = exp[log_e(e_i) + \beta_0 + \beta_1 X_{i1} + \ldots + \beta_p X_{ip}] \quad (6.2)$$

It is assumed that risk of an event rises directly with e_i and so in the model 6.2 the coefficient for $\log_e (e_i)$ is fixed at 1. This is known as an *offset* and is a special type of independent variable whose regression coefficient is fixed at unity. The values of e_i can be simply counts, person-years at risk or expected values.

Note that, as for the logistic regression, the *observed counts* have not yet appeared in the model. They are linked to the expected counts by the Poisson distribution (see Appendix 2). Thus, we assume that the observed count y_i is distributed as a Poisson variable with parameter $E_i = \lambda_i e_i$.

Instead of a measure of the person-years at risk, we could use the predicted number of deaths, based on external data. For example, we could use the age/sex specific death rates for England and Wales to predict the number of deaths in each group. This would enable us to model the *standardised mortality ratio* (SMR). For further details see Breslow and Day.[2] In other cases the e_i could simply be the denominator of a proportion.

Consider a cohort study in which the independent variable is a simple binary 0 or 1, respectively, for people not exposed or exposed to a hazard. The dependent variable is the number of people who succumb to disease during follow-up and also included in the model is the length of time they were on the study. Then, the coefficient b estimated from the model is the log of the ratio of the estimated incidence of the disease in those exposed and not exposed. Thus, exp(b) is the estimated *incidence rate ratio* (IRR) or *relative risk*. Note that for prospective studies the relative risk is a more natural parameter than an odds ratio (OR), particularly if the number of events is a high proportion of the number of subjects. One can also use Poisson regression when the outcome is binary, in other words when the data can be summarised in a 2×2 table relating input to output. The structure of the model is such that exp(b) still estimates the relative risk, without invoking the Poisson assumption. However, as the Poisson assumption is not met, the standard errors (SEs) are incorrect. Zou demonstrated a method of obtaining valid estimates using *robust SEs*.[3,4]

6.3 Interpreting a Computer Output: Poisson Regression

The data layout is exactly the same as for the grouped logistic regression described in Chapter 3. The model is fitted by maximum likelihood.

In 1951, Doll and Hill sent a questionnaire on smoking habits to 59,600 men and women on the British Medical Register. Responses were received from 34,445 men and 6192 women. The doctors were followed up over time and the underlying cause of death was collected from official death certificates. The data in Table 6.1 gives data on coronary deaths

Table 6.1 Coronary deaths from British male doctors.

Deaths (D)	Person-years	Smoker	Age group at start study	Expected (E)	$\frac{(D-E)}{\sqrt{E}}$
32	52,407	1	35–44	27.2	0.92
2	18,790	0	35–44	6.8	−1.85
104	43,248	1	45–54	98.9	0.52
12	10,673	0	45–54	17.1	−1.24
206	28,612	1	55–64	205.3	0.05
28	5712	0	55–64	28.7	−0.14
186	12,663	1	65–74	187.2	−0.09
28	2585	0	65–74	26.8	0.23
102	5317	1	75–84	111.5	−0.89
31	1462	0	75–84	21.5	2.05

and smoking among male doctors from the first ten years of the study quoted in Breslow and Day.[2,5] Here, the question is what is the risk of deaths associated with smoking, allowing for age? Thus, the dependent variable is number of deaths per age and per smoking group. Smoking group is the causal variable, age group is a confounder and the person-years is the offset. The expected values are given by the Poisson model. The computer analysis is given in Table 6.2.

The five age groups have been fitted using four dummy variables, with age group 35–44 as the reference group. The model used here assumes that the relative risk of coronary death for smokers remains constant for each age group. The first section of the output gives the coefficients for model 6.1 and the second part gives the exponentiated values, which are the IRRs or approximate relative risk The estimated relative risk for smokers compared to non-smokers is 1.43, with 95% confidence interval (CI) 1.16 to 1.76 which is highly significant ($P < 0.001$). Thus, male British doctors are 40% more likely to die of a coronary death if they smoke at each age group. An overall test of the model is the difference in deviances for the null and the model 935.064–12.133 = 922.931 which under the null hypothesis is distributed as a chi-squared distribution with 9–4 = 5 degrees of freedom (d.f.). This is very highly significant, but this significance is largely due to the age categories – coronary risk is highly age dependent. The test has five d.f. because there are five parameters in this particular model.

6.4 Model Checking for Poisson Regression

The simplest way to check the model is to compare the observed values and those expected by the model. The expected values are obtained by putting the estimated coefficients into Equation 6.2. Since the dependent variable is a count, we can use a chi-squared test to compare the observed and expected values and we obtain $X^2 = 12.13$, d.f. = 4, $p = 0.0164$. This is also given as the residual deviance in Table 6.2. This has four d.f. because the predicted

Table 6.2 Results of Poisson regression on data in Table 6.1.

```
Deviance Residuals:
       1        2       3        4       5        6        7       8
 0.90149 -2.17960 0.51023 -1.30766 0.05178- 0.13907 -0.08749 0.22928
       9       10
-0.91254  1.91944

Coefficients:
                Estimate  Std.  Error z value Pr(>|z|)
(Intercept)      -7.9194      0.1918 -41.298  < 2e-16
Smoker1           0.3546      0.1074   3.303 0.000957
Age.Group45-54    1.4840      0.1951   7.606 2.82e-14
Age.Group55-64    2.6275      0.1837  14.301  < 2e-16
Age.Group65-74    3.3505      0.1848  18.130  < 2e-16
Age.Group75-84    3.7001      0.1922  19.249  < 2e-16
---

(Dispersion parameter for poisson family taken to be 1)

    Null deviance: 935.064  on  9  degrees of freedom
Residual deviance:  12.133  on  4  degrees of freedom
AIC: 79.201

Number of Fisher Scoring iterations: 4

# Extract IRRs and CIs for Smoker and Age Group

                      IRR       2.5 %     97.5 %
Smoker1          1.425664   1.155102  1.759600
Age.Group45-54   4.410560   3.008998  6.464955
Age.Group55-64  13.838494   9.653850 19.837051
Age.Group65-74  28.516563  19.851637 40.963592
Age.Group75-84  40.451044  27.753174 58.958553
```

values are constrained to equal the observed values for the five age groups and one smoking group (the other smoking group constraint follows from the previous age group constraints). Thus, six constraints and ten observations yield four d.f. There is some evidence that the model does not fit the data. The deviance residuals are shown in Table 6.1. We expect most to lie between −2 and + 2 if there are no outliers and in fact only one value exceeds this. We can conclude there is little evidence of a systematic lack of fit of the model, except possibly for the non-smokers in the age group 75–84 years, but this is not a large difference.

The only additional term we have available to fit is the smoking × age interaction. This yields a saturated model (i.e. one in which the number of parameters equals the number of data points, see Appendix 2), and its likelihood ratio (LR) chi-squared is equal to the lack of fit chi-squared above. Thus, there is some evidence that smoking affects coronary risk differently at different ages.

6.5 Extensions to Poisson Regression

In the same way that the Binomial distribution defines the variance, so does the Poisson distribution. This means that Poisson models can have over-dispersion, in the same way that logistic models do. This is known as *extra-Poisson variation*. This is similar to *extra-Binomial variation* described in Chapter 3. The output in Table 6.2 contains the statement: '*Dispersion parameter for poisson family taken to be 1*'. This means that the SEs given assume the Poisson model. If over-dispersion occurs it means that the SEs given by the computer output may not be valid. It may arise because an important covariate is omitted. Another common situation which leads to over-dispersion is when the counts are correlated. This can happen when they refer to counts *within* an individual, such as number of asthma attacks per year, rather than counts within groups of separate individuals. This leads to a random effect model as described in Chapter 5, which, as explained there, will tend to increase our estimate of the SE relative to a model ignoring the random effect. Some packages now allow one to fit random effect Poisson models. A particular model that allows for extra variation in the λ_is is known as the *Negative Binomial regression* and this is available in R and other packages. If we think of the Binomial distribution P(x|n,p) as giving the probability of x successes out of n trials where each trial has probability p of success, the Negative Binomial distribution gives the probability of n trials, given that we require x successes. The reason for its name is that it can be shown that this probability is given by a Binomial distribution where some of the parameters are negative.

A further extension is when there are more zeros than would be expected by a Poisson distribution. For example, one might presume that the number of fish caught by different boats in a fishing trip would have a Poisson distribution (no joke intended), but if some boats had no rods, then they would inflate the number of zero counts. These models are called *zero-inflated* Poisson (ZIP) models and they are easily fitted with standard software.

Poisson regression is also used to calculate SMRs. Here the observed deaths O are assumed to have a Poisson distribution around the expected deaths E. The expected deaths are calculated using age/sex mortality tables. They are included in the model as an *offset* as described above.

6.6 Poisson Regression Used to Estimate Relative Risks from a 2 × 2 Table

Consider again Table 3.2. Rather than the OR, we wish to estimate the *relative risk* of death on Isoniazid compared to placebo.

We set up the data as shown in Table 3.2 for the ungrouped analysis. We are assuming that all subjects are followed up for the same length of time. We fit a Poisson model but use a "robust SE" estimator (to be specific HC3, see Appendix A3) to correct the SE because the Poisson assumption is invalid. The output is shown in Table 6.3, where the relative risk is described as the IRR. As described in Chapter 3, this is estimated as (11/132)/(21/131) = 0.52 which is the value shown in Table 6.3. The advantage of this method is that we can obtain valid estimates of the CI for the relative risk. These are given as 0.26 to 1.04, which correspond to those given in *Statistics at Square One* (Chapter 7). With robust SEs the Wald test

Table 6.3 Using Poisson regression to estimate a relative risk, as a substitute for logistic regression.

```
Coefficients:
               Estimate  Std. Error  z value Pr(>|z|)
(Intercept)   -1.83067     0.20150  -9.0852  < 2e-16
Treatment1    -0.65423     0.35386  -1.8489  0.06448

# Calculate IRR and 95% CI for Treatment

    IRR   2.5 % 97.5 %
  0.520   0.260  1.040
```

gives a *p*-value of 0.0645, which is somewhat larger than that given by the Wald test using logistic regression of 0.0602 in Table 3.3.

As Chapter 10 in *Statistics at Square One* explains, there are a wide variety of p-values for these data, depending on the test and the ones obtained here fit within the range given earlier. Using robust methods tends to give "conservative" p-values, that is, one rather larger than those obtained with more explicit assumptions.

6.7 Poisson Regression in the Medical Literature

Campbell *et al.*[6] looked at deaths from asthma over the period 1980–1995 in England and Wales. They used Poisson regression to test whether there was a trend in the deaths over the period, and concluded that, particularly for the age group 15–44, there had been a decline of about 6% (95% CI 5 to 7) per year since 1988, but this downward trend was not evident in the elderly.

Comment

This paper was a "short report" and so details of the model are not given. Since Poisson regression is a log-linear model, the slope is the percentage change from one year to the next. The authors included a quadratic term in the model to see if that improved the fit. The quadratic term was statistically significant, but the authors concluded that the linear model summarized the results well enough. It is always worth considering if trends over time are likely to be log-linear over the period of time considered, since they cannot go on for ever.

6.8 Ordinal Regression

When the outcome variable is *ordinal* then the methods described in the earlier chapters are inadequate. One solution would be to dichotomise the data and use logistic regression as discussed in Chapter 3. However, this is inefficient and possibly biased if the point for the dichotomy is chosen by looking at the data. The main model for ordinal regression is known as the *proportional odds* or *cumulative logit model.* It is based on the cumulative response probabilities rather than the category probabilities.

For example, consider an ordinal outcome variable Y with k ordered categorical outcomes y_j denoted by $j = 1, 2, ..., k$, and let $X_1, ..., X_p$ denote the covariates. The cumulative logit or proportional odds model is:

$$\text{logit}(C_j) = \log_e\left[\frac{C_j}{1-C_j}\right] = \log_e\left[\frac{\Pr(Y \le y_j)}{(\Pr(Y > y_j)}\right] = \alpha_i + \beta_1 X_1 + \cdots + \beta_p X_p \quad (6.3)$$

$$j = 1, 2, \ldots, k-1$$

or equivalently as:

$$\Pr(Y \le y_j) = \frac{\exp(\alpha_j + \beta_1 X_1 + \ldots + \beta_p X_p)}{1 + \exp(\alpha_j + \beta_1 X_1 + \ldots + \beta_p X_p)}, \ j = 1, 2, \ldots, k-1 \quad (6.4)$$

where $C_j = \Pr(Y \le y_j)$ is the cumulative probability of being in category j or less (note that for $j = k$; $\Pr(Y \le y_j|X) = 1$). Here, we have not used coefficients to indicate individuals to avoid cluttering the notation. Note that we have replaced the intercept term β_0 which would be seen in logistic regression by a set of variables, $\alpha_j, j = 1, 2, ..., k - 1$. When there are $k = 2$ categories, this model is identical to Equation 3.3, the logistic regression model. When there are more than two categories, we estimate separate intercepts terms for each category except the base category.

The regression coefficient β does not depend on the category j. This implies that the model 6.3 assumes that the relationship between the covariates X and Y is independent of j (the response category). This assumption of identical log ORs across the k categories is known as the *proportional odds assumption*.

The proportional odds model is useful when one believes the dependent variable is continuous, but the values have been grouped for reporting. Alternatively, the variable is measured imperfectly by an instrument with a limited number of values. The divisions between the boundaries are sometimes known as *cut points*. The proportional odds model is invariant when the codes for the response Y are reversed (i.e. y_1 recoded as y_k, y_2 recoded as y_{k-1} and so on). Second, the proportional odds model is invariant under the collapsibility of adjacent categories of the ordinal response (e.g. y_1 and y_2 combined and y_{k-1} and y_k combined).

Note that count data, described under Poisson regression, could be thought of as ordinal. However, ordinal regression is likely to be inefficient in this case because count data form a ratio scale and this fact is not utilised in ordinal regression (see Section 1.1).

The interpretation of the model is exactly like that of logistic regression. Continuous and nominal covariates can be included as independent variables.

6.9 Interpreting a Computer Output: Ordinal Regression

Consider a randomised controlled trial of health promotion in general practice to change people's eating habits, described in *Statistics at Square One*. Table 6.4 gives the results from a review at two years, to look at the change in the proportion of people eating poultry in those who had the health promotion literature (intervention) and those that did not (control).[7] Here there is a definite ordering of the outcome variable.

Table 6.4 Change in eating poultry in randomised trial.[7]

	Intervention	Control	Total	Proportion in intervention
	a	b	n	p = a/n
Increase	100	78	178	0.56
No change	175	173	348	0.50
Decrease	42	59	101	0.42
Total	317	310	627	0.51

Data from [8].

The outcome variable is now *ordinal* and it would be sensible to use an analysis that reflects this. In *Statistics at Square One* the analysis was done using a non-parametric Mann–Whitney *U*-test. Ordinal regression is equivalent to the Mann–Whitney test when there is only one binary independent variable 0/1 in the regression. The advantage of ordinal regression over non-parametric methods is that we get an efficient estimate of a regression coefficient and we can extend the analysis to allow for other confounding variables.

For the analysis, we coded the intervention as 1 and control as 0. The dependent variable was coded 1 (decrease), 2 (no change), 3 (increase), but in fact many packages will allow any positive whole numbers. The computer analysis is given in Table 6.5.

The log OR for the group is 0.3571. A separate piece of code gives us the OR exp(0.3571) = 1.43 with associated CI 1.05 to 1.94 (these are Wald-based CIs). The interpretation is that participants in the intervention group have 1.4 × the odds of consuming more poultry compared to the participants in the control group.

Table 6.5 Results of ordinal regression on data in Table 6.4.

```
Location coefficients:

       Estimate Std. Error z value  Pr(>|z|)
Group1   0.3571     0.1554  2.2974  0.021598

No scale coefficients

Threshold coefficients:
    Estimate Std. Error  z value
1|2  -1.4794     0.1304 -11.3462
2|3   1.1137     0.1221   9.1187

log-likelihood: -610.7695
AIC: 1227.539
Condition number of Hessian: 7.383805

# Calculate odds ratio and 95% CI

             OR     2.5 %    97.5 %
Group1 1.429212 1.053849 1.9382740
```

The threshold coefficients labelled 1 × 2 and 2 × 3 in the output are the two intercepts. They are known as ancillary parameters, meaning that they are extra parameters introduced to fit the model, but not part of the inferential study.

Useful discussions of the proportional odds model and other models for ordinal data have been given by Armstrong and Sloan,[8] Ananth and Kleinbaum[9] and Lall *et al.*[10] An excellent blog post has been given by Frank Harrell (https://www.fharrell.com/post/rpo). Harrell points out that when the proportional odds assumption does not hold, the OR from the proportional odds model represents a kind of average OR, and so can still have a useful interpretation. There is an almost one-to-one relationship between the OR and the concordance probability (which is a simple transformation of the Wilcoxon statistic). He states that a unified proportional odds model analysis is better than using inefficient and arbitrary analyses of dichotomized values of the independent variable.

Other models include the *continuation ratio model*, which considers the odds between two adjacent strata to be fixed, rather than the cumulative odds, but this is less frequently used. Armstrong and Sloan[8] concluded that the gain in efficiency using a proportional odds model as opposed to logistic regression is often not great, especially when the majority of the observations fall in one category. The strategy of dichotomising an ordinal variable and using logistic regression is simpler and easier to interpret, but can lead to loss of power and so some sensitivity analysis should be done. However, it is very important that the point of dichotomy is chosen *a priori* and not after having inspected several choices and choosing the one that conforms most closely to our prejudices. When there are a large number of categories it may be worth considering linear regression.

6.10 Model Checking for Ordinal Regression

Tests are available for proportional odds but these tests lack power. Also, the model is robust to mild departures from the assumption of proportional odds. A crude test would be to examine the ORs associated with each cut point. If they are all greater than unity, or all less than unity, then a proportional odds model will suffice.

From Table 6.4 we find the odds are:

Increase vs No change or decrease	Increase or No change vs Decrease
$OR = \frac{100 \times 232}{217 \times 78} = 1.37$	$OR = \frac{275 \times 59}{42 \times 251} = 1.54$

These ORs are quite close to each other and we can see that the observed OR of 1.43 from the proportional odds model is between the two. Thus we have no reason to reject the proportional odds model. Experience has shown that provided the odds do not actually change direction (e.g. the odds are all on the same side of unity) then the proportional odds model is pretty robust.[10]

Model testing is much more complicated when there is more than one input variable and some of them are continuous; specialist help should be sought.

6.11 Ordinal Regression in the Medical Literature

Hotopf *et al.*[11] looked at the relationship between chronic childhood abdominal pain as measured on three consecutive surveys at ages 7, 11 and 15 years and adult psychiatric disorders at the age of 36 years, in a cohort of 3637 individuals. A seven-point index of psychiatric disorder (the "index of definition") was measured as an outcome variable. This is an ordinal scale. It was found that the binary predictor (causal) variable, pain on all three surveys, was associated with an OR of 2.72 (95% CI 1.65 to 4.49) when potential confounder's sex, father's social class, marital status at age 36 years and educational status were included in the model. Thus, the authors conclude that children with abdominal pain are more likely to present psychiatric problems in later life. The usual cut-off for the index of definition is 5, but use of the whole scale uses more information and so gives more precise estimates.

6.12 Reporting the Results of Poisson or Ordinal Regression

- If the dependent variable is a count, then Poisson regression may be the required model. Give evidence that the model is a reasonable fit to the data by quoting the goodness-of-fit chi-squared. Test for covariate interaction or allow for extra-Poisson variation if the model is not a good fit.
- If the dependent variable is ordinal, then ordinal regression *may* be useful. However, if the ordinal variable has a large number of categories (say, > 7) then linear regression may be suitable. Give evidence that the proportional odds model is a reasonable one, perhaps by quoting the ORs associated with each cut point for the main independent variable. If proportional odds assumption is unlikely, then dichotomise the dependent variable and use logistic regression. *Do not* choose the point for dichotomy by choosing the one that gives the most significant value for the primary independent variable.

6.13 Reading about the Results of Poisson or Ordinal Regression

- As usual, look for evidence that the model is reasonable. In a Poisson model is there evidence of over-dispersion and, if so, has this been allowed for (i.e. by fitting a negative binomial regression model)?
- In Poisson regression, are the events making up the counts independent? If not, should over-dispersion be considered, for example by fitting a negative binomial model or a random effects model?
- If ordinal regression has been used are the cut-offs reasonable, for example standard definitions of a point which defines a clinically important outcome?
- Is the proportional odds model appropriate? Are the individual ORs between cut-off points similar?

6.14 Frequently Asked Question

Ordinal or Poisson regression?
There are occasions when the data are counts, but unlikely to come from a Poisson distribution. For example, a questionnaire might ask how many exacerbations in asthma has a patient had in the last month. This could range from 0 to 31. In this case it is unlikely that the data are distributed either as a Poisson or a Normal. The first action would be to tabulate the data. If most of the results were zero, then a logistic regression (exacerbations yes/no) would capture most of the information in the data. One certainly would not fit a zero inflated Poisson model. However, if the data distribution is, say, multimodal, with some having no exacerbations, some a few and some a lot, then an ordinal model, with sensible cut-offs, might give a more accurate picture of the outcome.

6.15 Exercises

Exercise 6.1

Stene *et al.*[12] looked at all live births in Norway from 1974 to 1998 and found 1828 children diagnosed with diabetes between 1989 and 1998. They fitted a Poisson regression model to the number of incident cases (D_j) and the person-time under observation (T_j) in each exposure category *j*. All confounders, such as maternal age and period of birth, were categorised. They investigated the relationship between birth weight and incidence of type 1 diabetes and found an almost linear relationship. They tested for interactions between birth weight and different categories of gestational age and found no interaction. In terms of model fit, they showed a graph of incidence of diabetes vs birth weight and stated that they tested for interactions.

a) Why were the potential confounders categorised?
b) If a graph of incidence of diabetes vs birth weight shows a straight line, is this reflected by the model?
c) What other tests of the model might one employ?
d) What other statistical models might be appropriate here?

Exercise 6.2

Wight *et al.*[13] carried out a survey of 3665 boys and 3730 girls aged under 16 years of age in Scotland. The main question was about sexual intercourse; 661 boys and 576 girls admitted to having had sex. The main outcome was whether their first time was "at the right age" (55% girls, 68% boys), "too early" (32% girls, 27% boys) or "should not have happened" (13% girls, 5% boys). The authors were interested in the effect of gender on this outcome, and whether the outcome was affected by social class and parenting style. The authors used ordinal regresson to analyse the data.

a) What type of variable is the outcome variable?
b) Describe what type of model is used to fit to this outcome, how it might be better than logistic regression and how a multivariate model could be used to adjust for social class and parenting style.

c) Discuss the assumptions for the model and give an informal check for the effect of gender on the outcome.

References

1 Clayton D, Hills M. *Statistical Models in Epidemiology*. Cary, North Carolina: Oxford University Press, 2013.

2 Breslow NE, Day NE. *Statistical Methods in Cancer Research: Vol II — The Design and Analysis of Cohort Studies*. Lyon: IARC, 1987.

3 Zou G. A modified Poisson regression approach to prospective studies with binary data. *Am J Epidemiol* 2004; **159**: 702–06.

4 Mansournia MA, Nazemipour M, Naimi AI, Collins GS, Campbell MJ. Reflections on modern methods: demystifying robust standard errors for epidemiologists. *Int J Epidemiol* 2021; 346–51. doi: 10.1093/ije/dyaa260

5 Doll R, Hill AB. Mortality of British doctors in relation to smoking: observations on coronary thrombosis. *Natl Cancer Inst Monog* 1996; **19**: 205–68.

6 Campbell MJ, Cogman GR, Holgate ST, Johnston SL. Age specific trends in asthma mortality in England and Wales 1983–1995: results of an observational study. *Br Med J* 1997; **314**: 1439–41.

7 Cupples ME, McKnight A. Randomised controlled trial of health promotions in general practice for patients at high cardiovascular risk. *BMJ* 1994; **309**: 993–96.

8 Armstrong BG, Sloan M. Ordinal regression models for epidemiologic data. *Am J Epidemiol* 1989; **129**: 191–204.

9 Ananth CV, Kleinbaum DG. Regression models for ordinal responses: a review of methods and applications. *Int J Epidemiol* 1997; **26**: 1323–33.

10 Lall R, Walters SJ, Campbell MJ, Morgan K, MRC CFAS. A review of ordinal regression models applied on health related quality of life assessments. *Stat Meth Med Res* 2002; **11**: 49–66.

11 Hotopf M, Carr S, Magou R, Wadsworth M, Wessely S. Why do children have chronic abdominal pain and what happens to them when they grow up? Population based cohort study. *Br Med J* 1998; **316**: 1196–200.

12 Stene LC, Magnus P, Lie RT, *et al.* Birth weight and childhood onset type I diabetes: population based cohort study. *Br Med J* 2001; **322**: 889–92.

13 Wight D, Henderson M, Raab G, *et al.* Extent of regretted sexual intercourse among young teenagers in Scotland: a cross-sectional survey. *Br Med J* 2000; **320**: 1243–44.

7

Meta-analysis

Summary

A meta-analysis is a statistical method that combines the results of multiple studies, initially trials but increasingly also observational studies. Meta-analysis can be performed when there are a number of scientific studies addressing the same question, with each individual study reporting the same outcomes. The aim is to derive a pooled estimate closest to the unknown common parameter. This chapter will discuss fixed and random effects models for meta-analysis, displaying data using a forest plot and the problems of missing studies and the use of a funnel plot. The controversy over fixed and random effect models is highlighted with an example.

7.1 Introduction

The idea that different studies looking at the same problem with quantitative outcomes could be combined is due to Glass,[1] who coined the term "meta-analysis" to describe the technique. In medicine, Archie Cochrane was an influential chest doctor and epidemiologist whose 1971 book: *Effectiveness and Efficiency*[2] strongly criticized the lack of reliable evidence behind many of the commonly accepted health care interventions at the time. His criticisms spurred rigorous evaluations of health care interventions and highlighted the need for evidence in medicine. He called for a systematic collection of studies, particularly randomised controlled trials, and this led to the creation of the Cochrane Collaboration which is a useful source of information on meta-analysis and provides a free program, "RevMan", for doing meta-analysis.[3]

In the age of reproducible results, the outcome from a single randomised trial is unlikely to change much clinical practice. Often there will be a number of trials looking at, say, the effectiveness of a particular treatment, and the question arises as to how to combine them.

The *Cochrane Handbook*[3] states that the main reasons for doing a meta-analysis are:

1) *To improve precision*. Many studies are too small to provide convincing evidence about intervention effects in isolation. Estimation is usually improved when it is based on more information.

Statistics at Square Two: Understanding Modern Statistical Application in Medicine, Third Edition.
Michael J. Campbell and Richard M. Jacques.

2) *To answer questions not posed by the individual studies.* Primary studies often involve a specific type of participant and explicitly defined interventions. A collection of studies in which these characteristics differ can allow investigation of the consistency of effect across a wider range of populations and interventions. It may also, if relevant, allow reasons for differences in effect estimates to be investigated.
3) *To settle controversies arising from apparently conflicting studies or to generate new hypotheses.* Statistical synthesis of findings allows the degree of conflict to be formally assessed, and reasons for different results to be explored and quantified.

A key benefit of this approach is the aggregation of information, leading to a higher statistical power and more robust point estimates than is possible from the measure derived from any individual study. However, in performing a meta-analysis, an investigator must make choices which can affect the results, including deciding how to search for studies, selecting studies based on a set of objective criteria, dealing with incomplete data and analysing the data. Judgement calls made in completing a meta-analysis may affect the results.

Meta-analyses are often, but not always, important components of a systematic review. For instance, a meta-analysis may be conducted on several clinical trials of a medical treatment in an effort to obtain a better understanding of how well the treatment works. Here it is convenient to follow the terminology used by the Cochrane Collaboration, and use "meta-analysis" to refer to statistical methods of combining evidence, leaving other aspects of "evidence synthesis", such as combining information from qualitative studies, for the more general context of systematic reviews. Although meta-analyses are often associated with combining clinical trials, it is possible to combine observational studies as well, and there exists a highly cited guideline for these (MOOSE).[4] However, due to the greater possibilities of bias, and natural differences in different observational studies, meta-analysis of observational data should be undertaken with care.[5]

In addition to the *Cochrane Handbook*,[3] which explains how to do meta-analysis with a variety of outcome measures, useful books on the subject are Borenstein *et al.*,[6] Whitehead[7] and Harrer *et al.*[8] The latter is freely available online. It gives an elementary introduction to meta-analysis and the R library *meta*.

7.2 Models for Meta-analysis

Methods for meta-analysis yield a weighted average from the results of the individual studies; what differs between methods is the manner in which these weights are allocated and also the manner in which the uncertainty is computed around the point estimate.

There are two sorts of meta-analysis: (1) one which uses individual patient data and (2) one which uses some summary measure, such an odds ratios (OR), a relative risk (RR) or an incidence rate ratio (IRR) of the same outcome from different studies. For continuous variables one can also use the standardised mean difference (SMD) which combines studies which have different continuous outcomes and derives a standardised effect by dividing the observed effect (e.g. difference between treatment and control) by the standard deviation of this difference. The summary measure approach is more common, since access to individual data from a number of studies is rare, and so this is the one we describe here.

Whatever the outcome, such as a log(OR) or a log(HR) the data for a meta-analysis comprise a measure y_i with standard error SE_i for each trial i, i = 1,...,k. In most meta-analyses the standard errors are assumed known and usually the *precision* or weight $w_i = 1/SE_i^2$ is used in the formulae. Note that SE_i^2 is inversely proportional to some measure of the sample size of the study and so w_i is a measure of the size of the study (e.g. for a two sample t-test with two groups of size n_1 and n_2, w_i is proportional to $n_1n_2/(n_1 + n_2)$ and so when $n_1 = n_2 = n$ it becomes n/2).

Consider a simple model in which there are k trials and each trial, i, is based on a treatment effect θ_i which comes from a distribution centred on the main effect, θ. A simple fixed effects model is:

$$y_i = \theta + \varepsilon_i \tag{7.1}$$

where ε_i is usually assumed to be Normally distributed with variance σ^2.

A weighted average is defined as:

$$\bar{y}_{\text{fix}} = \frac{\sum y_i w_i}{\sum w_i} \tag{7.2}$$

where w_i is the weight given to study i and the summation is over all studies.

Some simple algebra gives:

$$Var(\bar{y}_{\text{fix}}) = Var(\hat{\theta}) = \frac{1}{\sum w_i}$$

The assumption that the y_i come from the same population can be tested by the heterogeneity statistic:

$$Q = \sum w_i (y_i - \bar{y}_{\text{fix}})^2$$

Inside the summation sign we have a quantity (O - E)/SE(O). Under some general conditions this is approximately Normally distributed and the sum of its squares is approximately distributed as: χ^2_{k-1} The loss of one degree of freedom is for estimating the mean. In theory we can use Q as a test as to whether model (7.1) is true. However, care should be taken in the interpretation of the chi-squared test, since it has low power in the (common) situation of a meta-analysis when studies have small sample size or are few in number. This means that while a statistically significant result may indicate a problem with heterogeneity, a non-significant result must not be taken as evidence of no heterogeneity. This is also why a p-value of 0.10, rather than the conventional level of 0.05, is sometimes used to determine statistical significance, although in general a decision to use a random or fixed effects model based on the significance of the Q test is to be discouraged.

Consistency between studies can be measured using the I^2 statistic:

$$I^2 = \left(\frac{Q - (k-1)}{Q}\right) \times 100 \tag{7.3}$$

where *k - 1* is the degrees of freedom associated with Q.

If Q is less than $k - 1$ then I^2 is reported as zero. The logic behind I^2 is that if the estimates come from the same population then the expected value of Q is its degrees of freedom and so any excess could be due to heterogeneity. In general, trials are judged heterogeneous if I^2 is greater than 50%,[3] although as with any dichotomy this should not be an absolute rule.

Another measure is $H^2 = Q/(k-1)$ which is less commonly reported. Values of H^2 greater than one indicate between-study heterogeneity.

If the studies are heterogeneous then there are a number of options. The important starting point is explore the heterogeneity. This process can be problematic since there are often many characteristics that vary across studies from which one may choose. Heterogeneity may be explored by conducting subgroup analyses. However, explorations of heterogeneity that are devised after the heterogeneity is identified can at best lead to the generation of hypotheses. They should be interpreted with more caution and should generally not be listed among the conclusions of a review. Also, investigations of heterogeneity when there are very few studies are of questionable value. Another option is to perform a random-effects meta-analysis, which may be used to incorporate heterogeneity among studies. This is not a substitute for a thorough investigation of heterogeneity. It is intended primarily for heterogeneity that cannot be explained.

A simple random effects model is:

$$y_i = \theta + z_i + \varepsilon_i \tag{7.4}$$

Here z_i is a random term with expectation 0 and variance τ^2 which allows the between trial variability in the estimate of the treatment difference to be accounted for in the overall estimate and its SE. However, this assumes that the individual trials are in some way representative of what would happen in a population, even though centres taking part in trials are not chosen at random. In addition, if there are few trials in the meta-analysis, the estimate of τ^2 will be poor. In meta-analysis, random effects "allow for" heterogeneity but do not "explain" it. The weight used in Equation 7.2 is now: $w_i^* = \dfrac{1}{V_i + \widehat{\tau^2}}$ Again it can be shown that:

$$Var(\bar{y}_{\text{random}}) = Var(\hat{\theta}) = \frac{1}{\sum w_i^*} \tag{7.5}$$

We discussed the use of random effects models in cluster trials and repeated measures in Chapter 5.

Note that in a random effects model the link with the sample size is weakened. Suppose $\tau^2 = 0.1$ and $w_1 = 10$ and $w_2 = 100$. Then, using $V_i = 1/w_i$ we have $w_1^* = 1/(0.1 + 0.1) = 5$ and $w_2^* = 1/(0.01 + 0.1) = 9.1$. Thus, proportionately the larger trial gets a smaller weight.

There are a huge number of ways of estimating τ^2. The usual one is due to Dersimonian and Laird, but recently other measures using maximum likelihood and empirical Bayes procedures have been developed. Which estimator is best depends on a combination of the number of studies, the size or the studies and how much the size varies across studies.

The problem with confidence intervals (CI) is that they do not tell us what the range of estimates from future studies are likely to be (Julious *et al.*[9]) since they do not take into account the variability of future values. A problem with measures like τ^2 or I^2 is that their clinical interpretation is not straightforward. A prediction interval is less complicated; it presents the expected range of true effects in similar studies and can help in the interpretation of meta-analyses.[10]

Then an approximate 95% prediction interval is given by:

$$\hat{\theta} \pm t_{0.975,(k-1)}\sqrt{Var(\hat{\theta})}$$

This is called a prediction interval because it predicts the range of future values of θ and it is approximate because it doesn't taken into account the variability of the variance estimates. Bayesian methods can be used to allow for uncertainty in the variance estimates. It is, however, strongly based on the assumption of a Normal distribution for the effects across studies, and can be very problematic when the number of studies is small, in which case they can appear spuriously wide or spuriously narrow. It is useful when the number of studies is reasonable (e.g. more than ten) and there is no clear funnel plot asymmetry.

It is recommended that various methods should be used to explore heterogeneity. These include looking at subgroups, for example trials done in hospital compared to trials done outside, to see if within subgroups the results are heterogeneous. For individual patient data meta-analysis a technique known as *meta-regression* can be used to explore interactions between treatment effects and trial or patient characteristics.

7.3 Missing Values

Just as in standard data analysis, we should worry about missing data. In this case, the data that may be missing are *studies*. The most common reason why studies might be missing is because of so-called *publication-bias*. This can occur when studies which are not statistically significant are not written up and not published. Senn[11] argues this is not really a bias, since under the null hypothesis non-significant studies are equally likely to be in one direction as the other. However, bias can occur when a funder does not publish results which may adversely influence use of their product. *All trials*, a movement trying to get all trial results published has estimated that around 50% of trials are not published for various reasons.[12]

The simplest method of trying to detect if studies are missing is to search for trial protocols and then follow up to see if the main trial has been published. Some journals now require a pre-published protocol before they will accept the main trial for publication. There are a few statistical techniques for trying to see if the studies we have are plausibly representative and they are discussed below.

7.4 Displaying the Results of a Meta-analysis

The ways of displaying data in a meta-analysis are best described with an example. Gera and Sachdev[13] describe a meta-analysis of 29 trials of iron supplementation for the prevention of infections in children. The outcome measure is the IRR of infections in the treated group compared to the control (the IRR is the RR, discussed in Chapter 6).

An initial plot of the data should be a *forest plot* which is a plot of the estimates and CIs usually plotted vertically with each row a separate study, also referencing the study and the raw data. The forest plot for the data supplied by Gera and Sachdev[13] is given in Figure 7.1. Each CI is a measure of within-study variation; the wider CIs are associated with the smaller studies. The inverse variance weights are also given and one can see that the large study by Rice contributes 7.1% of the total weight whereas the tiny study by Nagpal with only six events contributes only 0.1% of the total weight. One would expect that omitting Nagpal's study would not change the results by much. One can see a wide variety of estimates, some favouring intervention and some not.

The test of heterogeneity Q, given at the bottom of the figure, is a test of whether the between- and within-study variation are commensurate. One can see from the p-value that they are not; there is more variation between studies than would be expected if they were all sampled from the same population. One can deduce that the I^2 statistic is $100 \times (78.29 - 28)/78.29 = 64\%$, indicating important heterogeneity since it is greater than 50%.

The pooled estimate using a random effects model is displayed in bold text at the bottom of the forest plot. In this case one can see that the CI includes unity, suggesting no real effect of iron supplementation on the incidence of infections.

The 95% prediction interval, the last CI on the plot, gives a range where we would expect the effect of similar future studies to lie based on the current evidence.

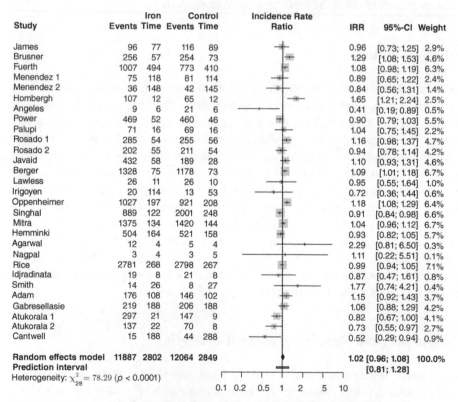

Study	Iron Events	Iron Time	Control Events	Control Time	IRR	95%-CI	Weight
James	96	77	116	89	0.96	[0.73; 1.25]	2.9%
Brusner	256	57	254	73	1.29	[1.08; 1.53]	4.6%
Fuerth	1007	494	773	410	1.08	[0.98; 1.19]	6.3%
Menendez 1	75	118	81	114	0.89	[0.65; 1.22]	2.4%
Menendez 2	36	148	42	145	0.84	[0.56; 1.31]	1.4%
Hombergh	107	12	65	12	1.65	[1.21; 2.24]	2.5%
Angeles	9	6	21	6	0.41	[0.19; 0.89]	0.5%
Power	469	52	460	46	0.90	[0.79; 1.03]	5.5%
Palupi	71	16	69	16	1.04	[0.75; 1.45]	2.2%
Rosado 1	285	54	255	56	1.16	[0.98; 1.37]	4.7%
Rosado 2	202	55	211	54	0.94	[0.78; 1.14]	4.2%
Javaid	432	58	189	28	1.10	[0.93; 1.31]	4.6%
Berger	1328	75	1178	73	1.09	[1.01; 1.18]	6.7%
Lawless	26	11	26	10	0.95	[0.55; 1.64]	1.0%
Irigoyen	20	114	13	53	0.72	[0.36; 1.44]	0.6%
Oppenheimer	1027	197	921	208	1.18	[1.08; 1.29]	6.4%
Singhal	889	122	2001	248	0.91	[0.84; 0.98]	6.6%
Mitra	1375	134	1420	144	1.04	[0.96; 1.12]	6.7%
Hemminki	504	164	521	158	0.93	[0.82; 1.05]	5.7%
Agarwal	12	4	5	4	2.29	[0.81; 6.50]	0.3%
Nagpal	3	4	3	5	1.11	[0.22; 5.51]	0.1%
Rice	2781	268	2798	267	0.99	[0.94; 1.05]	7.1%
Idjradinata	19	8	21	8	0.87	[0.47; 1.61]	0.8%
Smith	14	26	8	27	1.77	[0.74; 4.21]	0.4%
Adam	176	108	146	102	1.15	[0.92; 1.43]	3.7%
Gabresellasie	219	188	206	188	1.06	[0.88; 1.29]	4.2%
Atukorala 1	297	21	147	9	0.82	[0.67; 1.00]	4.1%
Atukorala 2	137	22	70	8	0.73	[0.55; 0.97]	2.7%
Cantwell	15	188	44	288	0.52	[0.29; 0.94]	0.9%
Random effects model	**11887**	**2802**	**12064**	**2849**	**1.02**	**[0.96; 1.08]**	**100.0%**
Prediction interval						**[0.81; 1.28]**	

Heterogeneity: $\chi^2_{28} = 78.29$ ($p < 0.0001$)

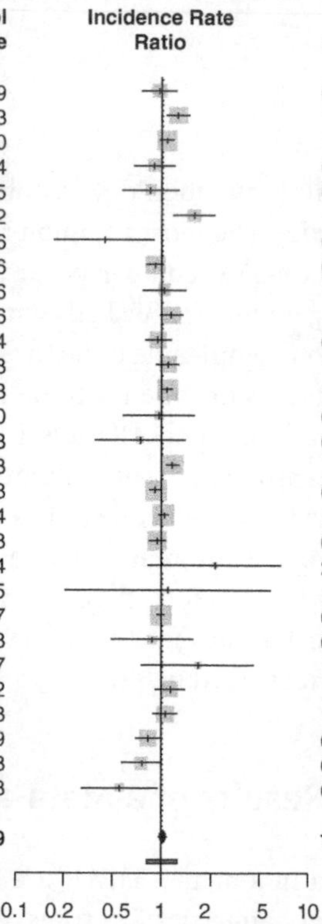

Figure 7.1 A forest plot for the incidence rate ratio for infection in 29 trials of iron supplementation in children for all infectious diseases.[13] Adapted from [13].

7.5 Interpreting a Computer Output

There are numerous programs for doing meta-analysis, including the Cochrane Collaboration RevMan. The results of analysing the data from Gera and Sachdev from the R library *meta*[8] are shown in Table 7.1. The analysis uses the option IRR and uses the log of the follow-up years as an offset. One can see that compared to the fixed effect the random effect estimate shrinks towards zero. The fixed effect IRR is 1.0217, whereas the random effect IRR is 1.0162. The default fitting method for the random effects model is REML (Restricted (or Residual) Maximum likelihood) which has been shown to perform better than older methods.[14] The I^2 and Q statistics suggest that a fixed effect model is untenable so one should report the random effect model as the main analysis. There is not much effect on the point estimate but the CI for the random effect is much wider, indicating the lower confidence in where the true result is, in view of the wide variety of observed risk ratios. The prediction interval shows the likely range of future trials, with IRRs from 0.81 to 1.28. Note that in fact five trials in the forest plot have estimated outcomes outside the 95% prediction interval, whereas one might have only expected one. It is unclear why this is so.

It should be noted that these effects can be obtained from Poisson regression as described in Chapter 6. For the fixed effect, we include 28 dummy variables for the studies and the results of an R fit are shown in Table 7.2. They are very close to the results given by *meta*.

Table 7.1 Analysis of data from Gera and Sachdev.

```
Number of studies combined: k = 29
Number of events: e = 23951

                          IRR             95%-CI     z  p-value
Common effect model    1.0217 [0.9957; 1.0483] 1.63   0.1021
Random effects model   1.0162 [0.9581; 1.0778] 0.53   0.5929
Prediction interval           [0.8053; 1.2823]

Quantifying heterogeneity:
 tau^2 = 0.0119 [0.0065; 0.0869]; tau = 0.1093 [0.0807; 0.2947]
 I^2 = 64.2% [46.9%; 75.9%]; H = 1.67 [1.37; 2.04]

Test of heterogeneity:
      Q d.f.  p-value
  78.29   28  < 0.0001

Details on meta-analytical method:
- Inverse variance method
- Restricted maximum-likelihood estimator for tau^2
- Q-profile method for confidence interval of tau^2 and tau
```

Table 7.2 Using Poisson regression to carry out a fixed effect analysis of data from Figure 7.1.

```
Deviance Residuals:
     Min         1Q     Median        3Q        Max
 -2.42865  -0.85621   0.00038   0.79806    2.25622

Coefficients:
             Estimate  Std. Error  z value  Pr(>|z|)
(Intercept)   0.23512     0.06895    3.410   0.00065    ***
Iron          0.02147     0.01308    1.641   0.10077


      IRR        2.5 %     97.5 %
1.021699   0.995838   1.048231
```

A useful plot to look for missing trials, and unusual ones, is a *funnel* plot. This is a plot of a measure of precision on the *y*-axis (the inverse of the SE, or the sample size), and a measure of effect on the *x*-axis (a difference in means, a log OR or a log risk ratio). If the studies are truly representative one would expect that the effect measures would be symmetrically distributed around a central point, so that small effects are as equally represented as large effects. The central point would have the highest precision so that the distribution would appear like an inverted funnel. An example of a funnel plot is given in Figure 7.2 from the study by Gera and Sachdev.[13] One can see that the plot is reasonably symmetrical and the studies with the highest precision (smallest SE) are clustered around the central value, which is close to 0. The authors concluded from this that there was little evidence of publication bias.

There are numerous statistical tests for asymmetry, such as that given by Egger and Davey-Smith,[15] but, as always, these tests should be used with caution and a non-significant result is not a guarantee of lack of bias, nor indeed a significant result a high degree of bias.

7.6 Examples from the Medical Literature

7.6.1 Example of a Meta-analysis of Clinical Trials

Zhang *et al.*[16] conducted a meta-analysis of trials of vitamin D supplementation and mortality. They found 50 trials with a total of 74,655 participants. They found no evidence of heterogeneity. Vitamin D supplementation was not associated with all-cause mortality (risk ratio 0.98, 95% CI 0.95 to 1.02, $I^2 = 0\%$), cardiovascular mortality (0.98, 95% CI: 0.88 to 1.08, $I^2 = 0\%$) or non-cancer, non-cardiovascular mortality (1.05, 95% CI: 0.93 to 1.18, $I^2 = 0\%$). Vitamin D supplementation statistically significantly reduced the risk of cancer death (0.85, 95% CI: 0.74 to 0.97, $I^2 = 0\%$). In subgroup analyses, all-cause mortality was significantly lower in trials with vitamin D_3 supplementation than in trials with vitamin D_2 supplementation (p-value for interaction = 0.04); neither

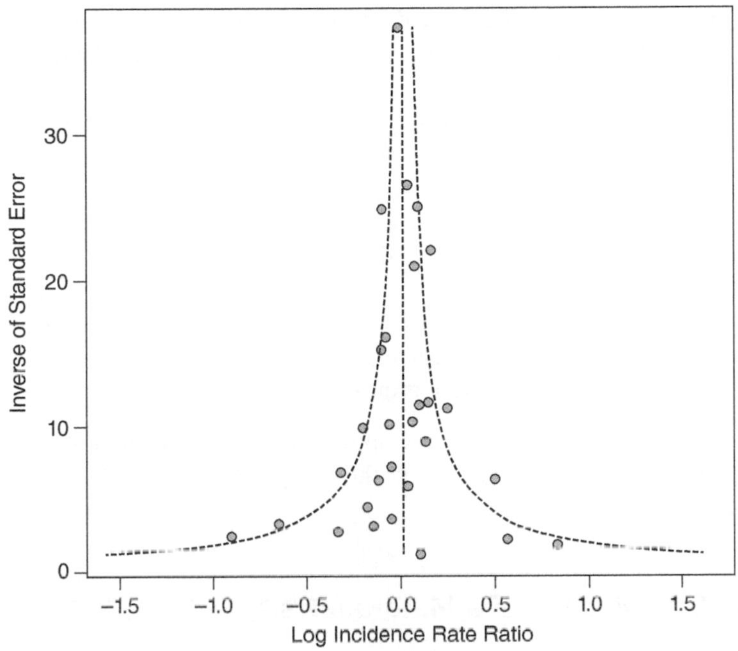

Figure 7.2 A funnel plot for the iron supplementation study of Gera and Sachdev.[13]
Gera T, Sachdev HP. Effect of iron supplementation on incidence of infectious illness in children: a systematic review. *BMJ* 2002; **325**: 1142–51. https://www.bmj.com/content/325/7373/1142

vitamin D_3 nor vitamin D_2 was associated with a statistically significant reduction in all-cause mortality.

7.6.2 Example of a Meta-analysis of Case-control Studies

An example of a meta-analysis, not of trials but of case-control studies, has already been described in Chapter 3 (Table 3.10).[17] It is analysed there as a fixed effects model. However, the four case-control studies described there could be regarded as four samples from a larger pool of potential case-control studies, and hence a random effects model may seem appropriate. Here the z_i term would reflect the heterogeneity of the intervention effect over studies.

7.7 Reporting the Results of a Meta-analysis

The Cochrane collaboration has a checklist for reporting systematic reviews, the Preferred Reporting Items for Systematic Reviews and Meta-Analysis (PRISMA), and part of this includes the reporting of meta-analysis.[18] (This was formerly known as the QUORUM statement.) The items include:

- If statistical synthesis methods were used, reference the software, packages and version numbers used to implement synthesis methods.

- Specify the meta-analysis model (fixed-effect, fixed-effects or random-effects) and provide rationale for the selected model and specify the method used (e.g. Mantel-Haenszel, inverse-variance).
- Specify any methods used to identify or quantify statistical heterogeneity (e.g. visual inspection of results, a formal statistical test for heterogeneity, heterogeneity variance (τ^2), inconsistency (e.g. I^2) and prediction intervals).
- If a random-effects meta-analysis model was used, specify the between-study (heterogeneity) variance estimator used (e.g. DerSimonian and Laird, REML).
- Specify the method used to calculate the CI for the summary effect (e.g. Wald-type CI).
- If methods were used to explore possible causes of statistical heterogeneity, specify the method used (e.g. subgroup analysis, meta-regression).
- Give an estimate of the absolute risks in different groups.

It is worth noting that the Cochrane Handbook[3] recommends that p-values are not used to decide statistical significance in meta-analysis and the main reporting should be the combined estimate and a CI.

7.8 Reading about the Results of a Meta-analysis

When reading a paper about meta-analysis one should go through the PRISMA statement and if items are not reported make a judgement as to whether these are likely to affect the conclusion.

Looking through the checklist for the paper by Zhang *et al.*,[16] one can see they did reference the software packages and version numbers used. They stated that they used fixed effects model if $I^2 < 50\%$ and otherwise random effects. They did not specify the heterogeneity variance estimator nor how the CIs were calculated, although, to be fair it would be easy to find out the methods from the package they used. They used both subgroup analysis and meta-regression to explore heterogeneity in particular, different cases of death and difference types of vitamin D.

In addition, one should use the skills learned earlier in this book for reading any scientific paper to critically appraise the paper. For example, there are at least four outcomes in Zhang *et al.*'s paper: total mortality, deaths from cancer, deaths from cardiovascular disease and non-cancer, non-cardiovascular disease, and yet only cancer mortality is statistically significant. This leads one to question whether one should simply use a significance test to decide that vitamin D protects against cancer death and also question whether the authors should have adjusted for multiple tests. In addition, only RR reduction is quoted. What is the absolute risk reduction for cancer mortality? Is it worth worrying about?

7.9 Frequently Asked Questions

1) *Should I use a fixed or random effects model in a meta-analysis?*
   There is much controversy in this area. The advice of Whitehead[7] (p. 153) (and many other authors) is that the choice should not be made solely on whether the

test for heterogeneity is significant. We need to consider additional criteria such as the number of trials, the relative size of the trials and the distribution of the summary measures. With a small number of trials it is difficult to estimate between trial variability; if the results from the trials appear consistent, then a fixed effects model may be more appropriate. If, however, there are a large number of trials and no very small trials, then a random effects model should be more generalisable. It may be useful to fit both, and if the heterogeneity is low, the effect estimates from the fixed and random models will agree. If the results differ, then further investigation is warranted. Some have argued that the name "fixed" effect is misleading; one can still get a valid estimate of an overall effect using a fixed effect model without having to invoke the assumption that the underlying risk is constant.[19] The random effect model gives less weight to individual deaths in large studies than in smaller ones, which can lead to discrepancies between fixed effect and random effects if there are many small trials and only a few large trials in the analysis. The CI for the random-effects meta-analysis reflects both the uncertainty in estimating the average treatment effect across trials and the uncertainty in estimating the between-trial variance; so when some trials are small this will be large. A case in point is the REACT meta-analysis of seven trials examining the association between systemic corticosteroids and 28-day mortality among critically ill patients with Covid-19.[20] They found a summary OR of 0.66 (95% CI 0.53 to 0.82) $P < 0.001$ using a fixed effect model and little heterogeneity. The random effects OR was 0.70 (95% CI 0.48 to 1.01) $P = 0.053$. The reason for this discrepancy in CIs is that the RECOVERY trial randomised 1007 patients whereas the other six trials randomised only 696 and so uncertainties in the estimates of the small trials affect the random effects CI. The authors had pre-specified the fixed effects model and concluded that administration of systemic corticosteroids, compared with usual care or placebo, was associated with lower 28-day all-cause mortality in critically ill patients with Covid-19. A pleasing point is that they also reported absolute risks, namely an approximate 32% mortality with corticosteroids compared with 40% with usual care or placebo.

2) *Are the results of a meta-analysis of trials higher in the hierarchy of scientific rigour than a randomised clinical trial?*
One would expect that since randomised clinical trials are supposed to be higher in the so-called hierarchy of scientific rigour (better than case reports, observational studies, case-control studies and non-randomised longitudinal studies) that meta-analysis would trump them all. However, it is important to recall that a meta-analysis is an analysis of observational data, which contains biases beyond the analysist's control, such as publication bias, and so meta-analysis should not be awarded the status of the final answer. Indeed it is not uncommon for meta-analyses in the same area to disagree.
3) *Are power calculations relevant to a meta-analysis?*
As mentioned in FAQ (2) meta-analyses are observational data and often the analyst has no control over the number of studies available. The minimum number of studies for a meta-analysis is two. One power calculation that is relevant is if one wants to conduct a new clinical trial, one can ask how big would it have to be to change the result of the most recent meta-analysis?

4) *Are there alternatives to weighting by the inverse of the variance?*
   For binary effect size data, there are alternative methods to calculate the weighted average, including the Mantel–Haenszel, Peto or a sample size weighting method.[6]

7.10 Exercise

Guilbert *et al.*[21] carried out a systematic review of short-term effectiveness of nutrition therapy to treat type 2 diabetes in low-income and middle-income countries. They found two studies with outcomes at three months after the intervention and two studies with outcomes at six months. The results for changes in HbA1c are shown in Figure 7.3

Questions

1) What type of plot is Figure 7.3?
2) Are the outcomes different for three months and six months?
3) Why is the I^2 statistic 0 and the H^2 statistic 1, for the three-month outcome?
4) Is there evidence of heterogeneity within each time group and overall?
5) For the six-month outcome derive the I^2 and H^2 statistics from Q
6) Why are there three degrees of freedom associated with Q?

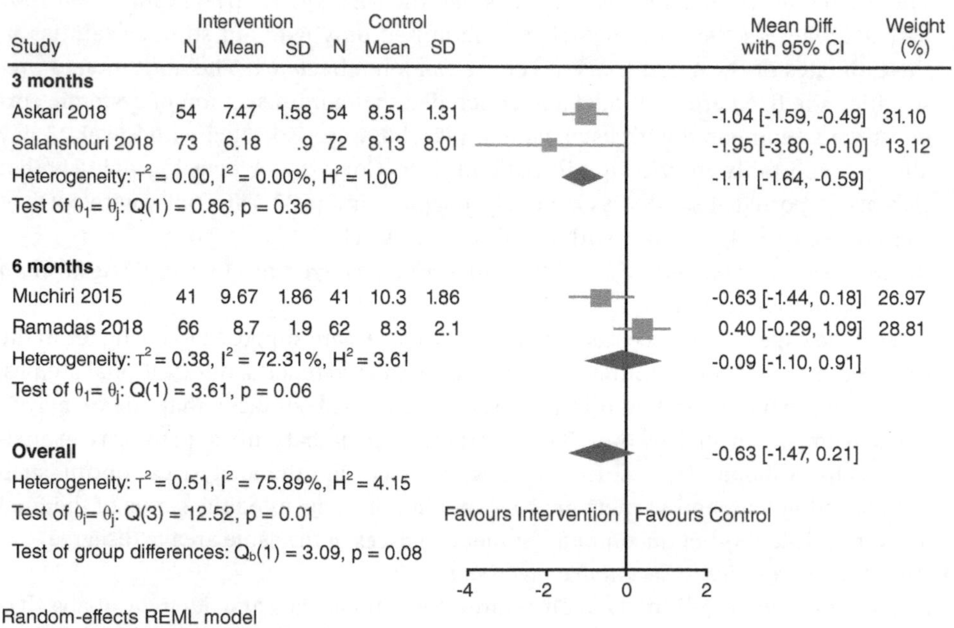

Figure 7.3 Results from four trials on nutritional therapy in Type 1 Diabetes: differences in mean HbA1c (Intervention - Control).

References

1 Glass GE. Primary, secondary and meta-analysis of research. *Educational Research* 1976; **5**: 3–8.

2 Cochrane AL. *Effectiveness and Efficiency (Nuffield Provincial Hospitals Trust)*. London: Burgess and Son Ltd, 1972.

3 Deeks JJ, Higgins JPT, Altman DG, *et al.* (eds.) Chapter 10: analysing data and undertaking meta-analyses. In: Higgins JPT, Thomas J, Chandler J, Cumpston M, Li T, Page MJ, Welch VA (editors). *Cochrane Handbook for Systematic Reviews of Interventions* version 6.3 (updated February 2022). Cochrane, 2022. Available from www.training.cochrane.org/handbook

4 Stroup DF, Berlin JA, Morton SC, *et al.* Meta-analysis of observational studies in epidemiology: a proposal for reporting. *JAMA* 2000; **283**(15): 2008–12.

5 Metelli S, Chaimani A. Challenges in meta-analyses with observational studies. *Evidence-Based Mental Health* 2020; **23**: 83–7.

6 Borenstein M, Hedges LV, Higgins JP, Rothstein HR. *Introduction to Meta-analysis*, 2nd edn. New York: John Wiley & Sons, 2021.

7 Whitehead A. *Meta-analysis of Controlled Clinical Trials*. Chichester: John Wiley, 2002.

8 Harrer M, Cuijpers P, Furukawa TA, Ebert DD. *Doing Meta-Analysis with R: A Hands-On Guide*. Boca Raton, FL and London: Chapman & Hall/CRC Press, 2021.

9 Julious SA, Campbell MJ, Walters SJ. Predicting where future means will lie based on the results of the current trial. *Contemporary Clinical Trials* 2007; **28**: 352–7.

10 IntHout J, Ioannidis JPA, Rovers MM, *et al.* Plea for routinely presenting prediction intervals in meta-analysis. *BMJ Open* 2016; **6**: e010247. doi: 10.1136/bmjopen-2015-010247

11 Senn S. *Chapter 16 Meta Analysis. In Statistical Issues in Drug Development*, 2nd edn. Chichester: Wiley, 2007.

12 All Trials Website. https://www.alltrials.net (accessed February 2022).

13 Gera T, Sachdev HP. Effect of iron supplementation on incidence of infectious illness in children: a systematic review. *BMJ* 2002; **325**: 1142–51.

14 Tanriver-Ayder E, Faes C, van de Casteele T, *et al.* Comparison of commonly used methods in random effects meta-analysis: application to preclinical data in drug discovery research. *BMJ Open Science* 2021; **5**: e100074. doi: 10.1136/bmjos-2020-100074

15 Egger M, Davey Smith G, Schneider M, Minder C. Bias in meta-analysis detected by a simple, graphical test. *BMJ* 1997; **315**: 629–34. doi: 10.1136/bmj.315.7109.629

16 Zhang Y, Fang F, Tang J, *et al.* Association between vitamin D supplementation and mortality: systematic review and meta analysis. *BMJ* 2019; **366**: l4673.

17 Wald NJ, Nanchahal K, Thompson SG, Cuckle HS. Does breathing other people's tobacco smoke cause lung cancer? *Br Med J* 1986; **293**: 1217–22.

18 Page MJ, McKenzie JE, Bossuyt PM, *et al.* The PRISMA 2020 statement: an updated guideline for reporting systematic reviews. *BMJ* 2021; **372**: n71. doi: 10.1136/bmj.n71

19 Rice K, Higgins JPT, Lumley T. A re-evaluation of fixed effect(s) meta-analysis. *J R Stat Soc Ser A (Stat Soc)* 2018; **181**: 205–27.

20 The WHO Rapid Evidence Appraisal for COVID-19 Therapies (REACT) Working Group. Association between administration of systemic corticosteroids and mortality among critically ill patients with COVID-19: a meta-analysis. *JAMA* 2020; **324**(13): 1330–41. doi: 10.1001/jama.2020.17023

21 Guilbert E, Perry R, Whitmarsh A, *et al.* Short-term effectiveness of nutrition therapy to treat type 2 diabetes in low income and middle-income countries: systematic review and meta-analysis of randomised controlled trials. *BMJ Open* 2022; **12**: e056108. doi: 10.1136/bmjopen-2021-056108

8

Time Series Regression

Summary

Time series regression is mainly used when the outcome is continuous, but measured together with the predictor variables serially over time. Possibly the most useful example is *interrupted time series*. When an intervention is given over an entire region the only option of evaluating the intervention is to compare results in time before and after the intervention. These are also called *discontinuity models*.

8.1 Introduction

Time series regression is concerned with the situation in which the dependent and independent variables are measured over time. Usually there is only a single series with one dependent variable and a number of independent variables, unlike repeated measures when there may be several series of data.

The potential for confounding in time series regression is very high – many variables either simply increase or decrease over time, and so will be correlated over time. In addition, many epidemiological variables are seasonal, and this variation would be present even if the factors were not causally related. It is important that seasonality and trends are properly accounted for. Simply because the outcome variable is seasonal, it is impossible to ascribe causality because of seasonality of the predictor variable. For example, sudden infant deaths are higher in winter than in summer, but this does not imply that temperature is a causal factor; there are many other factors that might affect the result, such as reduced daylight, or presence of viruses. However, if an unexpectedly cold winter is associated with an increase in sudden infant deaths, or very cold days are consistently followed after a short time by rises in the daily sudden infant death rate, then causality may possibly be inferred.

Often when confounding factors are correctly accounted for, the serial correlation of the residuals disappears; they appear serially correlated because of the association with a time dependent predictor variable, and so conditional on this variable the residuals are independent. This is particularly likely for mortality data, where, except in epidemics, the

Statistics at Square Two: Understanding Modern Statistical Application in Medicine, Third Edition.
Michael J. Campbell and Richard M. Jacques.

individual deaths are unrelated. Thus, one can often use conventional regression methods followed by a check for the serial correlation of the residuals and need only proceed further if there is clear evidence of a lack of independence.

If the inclusion of known or potential confounders fails to remove the serial correlation of the residuals, then it is known that ordinary least squares does not provide valid estimates of the SEs of the parameters.

A very common use of time series methodology is in *interrupted time series*[1,2] or *discontinuity design*.[3] These are often used in public health where an intervention affects a complete community and so there is no possibility of a contemporaneous control, but one can compare data collected before and after the intervention (they are sometimes called "before-and-after" studies). The Covid epidemic produces many such possibilities. The main issues are how the intervention changes the outcome. It may have an immediate effect, it may change a trend or it may do both. The data are collected in time so the problem of serial correlation may exist or may be removed by modelling with time changing covariates.

8.2 The Model

For a continuous outcome, suppose the model is:

$$y_t = \beta_0 + \beta_1 X_{t1} + \ldots + \beta_p X_{tp} + v_t, t = 1,\ldots, n \tag{8.1}$$

The main difference from Equation 2.1 is that we now index time t rather than individuals. It is important to distinguish time points because whereas two individuals with the same covariates are interchangeable, you cannot swap, say Saturday with Sunday and expect the same results. We denote the error term by v_t and we assume that $v_t = \varepsilon_t - \alpha v_{t-1}$ where the ε_t are assumed independent Normally distributed variables with mean 0 and variance σ^2 and α is a constant between -1 and $+1$. The error term is known as an *autoregressive process (of order 1)*. This model implies that the data are correlated in time, known as *serial correlation*. The effect of ignoring serial correlation is to provide artificially low estimates of the SE of the regression coefficients and thus to imply significance more often than the significance level would suggest under the null hypothesis of no association.

For an interrupted times series it can help to redefine t so that $t = 0$ occurs at the time of the intervention (t_0); Define $\delta_t = 1$ when $t \geq 0$ and $= 0$ otherwise. A simple model for an interrupted time series is:

$$y_t = \beta_0 + \beta_1(1-\delta_t)t + \beta_2\delta_t + \beta_3\delta_t t + v_t, t = -t_0,\ldots, 0,\ldots, n - t_0 \tag{8.2}$$

where β_1 is the slope before the intervention, β_3 is the slope after the intervention and β_2 is the immediate effect of the intervention.

8.3 Estimation Using Correlated Residuals

Given the above models, and assuming α is known, we can use a method of generalised least squares known as the *Prais–Winsten / Cochrane–Orcutt procedure*.[4]

For simplicity assume one independent variable and write:

$$y_t^* = y_t - \alpha y_{t-1}$$

and:

$$x_t^* = X_t - \alpha X_{t-1}$$

We can then obtain an estimate of β using ordinary least squares on y_t^* and x_t^*. However, since α will not usually be known it can be estimated from the ordinary least squares residuals e_t by:

$$\hat{\alpha} = \frac{\sum_{t=2}^{n} e_t e_{t-1}}{\sum_{t=2}^{n} e_{t-1}^2}$$

One can test whether $\hat{\alpha}$ is significantly different from zero using what is known as the *Durbin–Watson* test.

This leads to an iterative procedure in which we can construct a new set of transformed variables and thus a new set of regression estimates and so on until convergence. The iterative Cochrane–Orcutt procedure can be interpreted as a stepwise algorithm for computing maximum likelihood estimators of α and β where the initial observation y_1 is regarded as fixed. If the residuals are assumed to be Normally distributed then full maximum likelihood methods are available, which estimate α and β simultaneously. This can be generalised to higher order autoregressive models and fitted in a number of computer packages. However, caution is advised in using this method when the autocorrelations are high, and it is worth making the point that an autoregressive error model should not be used as a nostrum for models that simply do not fit.

These models can be generalised to outcomes which are binary or counts, but this is beyond the scope of this book and for further details see Campbell.[5, 6]

In general, ordinary least squares produces unbiased estimates, so one approach to analysis is to use a robust standard error such as the Newey–West standard error to allow for both heterogeneous variance and autocorrelation. Details are given in Berger.[7]

8.4 Interpreting a Computer Output: Time Series Regression

Suppose that the data on deadspace and height in Table 2.1 in fact referred to one individual followed up over time. Then the regression of deadspace against height is given in Table 8.1 using Cochrane–Orcutt regression. This method loses the first observation, and so the regression coefficient is not strictly comparable with that from the linear regression model, not allowing for autocorrelation, but they are similar. Note that the output gives the number of degrees of freedom as 12, not 13, since one is used for the autocorrelation coefficient. Note also that the SE, 0.21, obtained from the Cochrane-Orcutt regression is much larger than the value 0.18 when all the points are assumed to be independent. The estimate of α (*rho*), the autocorrelation coefficient is denoted rho and is quite small at 0.0.046 and not significant ($p = 0.3$), as might be expected since the data are not, in fact, autocorrelated.

Table 8.1 Results of Cochrane–Orcutt regression of deadspace against height on the data in Table 2.1 assuming points all belong to one individual over time.

```
Analysis not allowing for autocorrelation

Coefficients:
             Estimate  Std. Error  t value   Pr(>|t|)
(Intercept) -82.4852      26.3015   -3.136    0.00788
Height        1.0333       0.1804    5.728   6.96e-05
---

Residual standard error: 13.07 on 13 degrees of freedom
Multiple R-squared:  0.7162,    Adjusted R-squared:  0.6944
F-statistic: 32.81 on 1 and 13 DF,  p-value: 6.956e-05

Analysis allowing for autocorrelation

rho 0.046349
                 Estimate     Std. Error  t value      Pr(>|t|)
(Intercept)    -102.11676       31.78251   -3.213     0.0074508
Height            1.16017        0.21439    5.412     0.0001571
---
Residual standard error: 12.8574 on 12 degrees of freedom
Multiple R-squared:  0.7093,    Adjusted R-squared:  0.6851
F-statistic: 29.3 on 1 and 12 DF,  p-value: < 1.571e-04

Durbin-Watson statistic
(original):     1.83407,  p-value: 2.599e-01
(transformed): 1.90158,  p-value: 3.032e-01>
```

8.5 Example of Time Series Regression in the Medical Literature

Arain *et al.*[8] describe a study of a general practitioner (GP) led "walk-in centre" which was introduced in Sheffield in 2011. A study was conducted to see if this would affect the number of attendances at the emergency department in the town. There was no control group, simply the monthly attendance figures at the emergency department before and after the start of the "walk-in centre". Potential confounding factors are seasonality and trend in the model. A model similar to Equation 8.2 was fitted, including dummy variables to model monthly effects. The walk-in centre was closed at night and so was not expected to affect the night-time emergency department attendances. These values could be used as a further covariate to control for external factors since they are likely to have the same trends as day.

The average number of monthly adult attendances in the year before the walk-in centre was set up was 2758 and after it was 2616. Allowing for seasonal variation and a time trend, this suggested a reduction of 230.9 attendances per month. Using the additional control variable of night-time attendances to allow for other external influences this reduced the effect size to 137.9. The residuals were plausibly independent, and the 95% confidence interval (CI) was 21.9 to 438.9, $p = 0.03$, giving some evidence for a small effect of the walk-in centre on attendances at the emergency department. If night-time attendances were used as a control, the effect on adult emergency department attendance was a 5% reduction (95% CI 1% to 9%).

8.6 Reporting the Results of Time Series Regression

The Equator network states that reporting guidelines for interrupted time series (FERITS) are under development.[9]

- Always include the fact that the data form a time series in the title.
- Give the test for autocorrelation and the autocorrelation coefficient.
- Describe the model. For an interrupted time series, is there a change in level, a change in slope or both?
- As stated in *Statistics at Square One*, there is something strange about doing a significance test to decide whether to fit a different model. It is probably better to give a model which does not allow for serial correlation and one that does and see what effect it has on interpretation

8.7 Reading about the Results of Time Series Regression

- If the model assumes linearity, has this been checked?
- Has allowance for autocorrelation been made?
- Look for evidence that the residuals in the model are serially correlated. If they are, then does the model allow for them?
- For an interrupted time series, how has time been defined and what are the interpretations of the intercept terms in the model?

8.8 Frequently Asked Questions

1) *Are there other models for autocorrelation besides an AR(1)?*
   It would appear that an assumption of an AR(1) model for time series is something like the assumption of proportional hazards for survival or equality of variance for continuous data; something which is tacitly assumed in most cases. In fact, there are a huge variety of autoregressive, integrated moving average models (ARIMA) which could be used, but are rarely needed. For example, Campbell[6] fitted an AR(7) to allow for a weekly correlation in daily sudden infant death rates.
2) *Should one always allow for autocorrelation in time series?*
   It is often the case that when using time dependent covariates in a model, the error terms are no longer serially correlated. If they are correlated it could be because the model does not fit (e.g. the relationship of the dependent variable with time is quadratic not linear). In general it is poor practice to use an autoregressive model simply to cover up a poor fitting model.

8.9 Exercise

Ballard *et al.*[10] assessed whether adequately supported community care workers (CHWs) could maintain the continuity of essential community-based health service provision during the Covid-19 pandemic. They looked at five regions in Africa. The pandemic was declared in March 2020 and so monthly health data from January 2018 to February 2020 were used as a baseline against which to compare utilisation rates for April–June 2021. The segmented linear regression model was:

$$Y_t = \beta_0 + \beta_1 \times \text{time} + \beta_2 \times \text{pandemic} + \beta_3 \times \text{post-slope} + \text{region} + \varepsilon_t$$

Where Y_t is the outcome variable at time t, time (in months) is a continuous variable indicating time from January 2018 up to June 2021. Pandemic (i.e. the Covid-19 pandemic) is coded 0 for pre-pandemic time points and 1 for post-pandemic time points, with March 2020 as null, while post-slope is coded 0 up to the last point before the pandemic phase and coded sequentially thereafter. Region is a dummy variable for each of the five regions.

Auto-correlation was controlled by performing a Durbin–Watson test to test the presence of first-order auto-correlation and because auto-correlation was detected, using the Prais–Winsten generalised least squares estimator to estimate the regression coefficients.

One of the outcomes used was iCCM Speed, which is the percentage of children under five assessed with a symptom of malaria, diarrhoea or pneumonia, within 24 hours of symptom onset each month. The results are shown in Table 8.2.

Comment

The authors reference the package R but do not say which libraries they used. They state they used a Durbin–Watson test but do not give the results. They gave graphs of the data, but did not check for linearity. They looked at alternative models such as excluding region from the model which did not affect the slopes. They did not centre time at the start of the intervention, which means that the estimate β_2 is the difference in the slopes in January 2018. They concluded there was a small decrease in the rate of iCCM Speed with time during the pandemic.

Table 8.2 Results of interrupted time series regression for iCCM Speed.[10]

Metric	Independent variables	Coefficient	SE	P-value
iCCM Speed	Constant (β0)	23.80	2.05	< 0.0001
	Time (β1)	0.48	0.11	< 0.0001
	Intervention (β2)	−1.62	2.11	0.44
	Post-slope (β3)	−0.69	0.28	0.0165
	Region 2	−4.33	0.85	< 0.000
	Region 4	55.24	0.86	< 0.0001

Data from [10]

Questions

1) What was the value of iCCM Speed in January 2018 in Region 1?
2) What is the predicted value of iCCM Speed in January 2019 (t = 13)?
3) What is the predicted iCCM Speed for Region 4 in January 2018?
4) What is the immediate effect on iCCM Speed when the pandemic was declared?
5) Is it assumed the Regions affect the slopes?
6) Why are Region 3 and Region 5 excluded from the model?

References

1 Bernal JL, Cummins S, Gasparrini A. Interrupted time series regression for the evaluation of public health interventions: a tutorial. *Int J Epidemiol* 2017; **46**(1): 348–55. doi: 10.1093/ije/dyw098 Erratum in: *Int J Epidemiol* 2020; **49**(4): 1414. PMID: 27283160; PMCID: PMC5407170.

2 López Bernal J. *The use of interrupted time series for the evaluation of public health interventions.* PhD (research paper style) thesis, London School of Hygiene & Tropical Medicine, 2018. https://doi.org/10.17037/PUBS.04648680

3 Venkataramani AS, Bor J, Jena AB. Regression discontinuity designs in healthcare research. *Br Med J* 2016; **352**: i1216. doi: 10.1136/bmj.i1216

4 Wooldridge JM. *Introductory Econometrics. A Modern Approach*, 5th edn. Mason, OH: South-Western Cengage Learning Cengage, 2013.

5 Campbell MJ. Article stat05541 Time series regression. Wiley Statistics Reference. 2016. https://doi.org/10.1002/9781118445112.stat05541.pub2

6 Campbell MJ. Time series regression for counts: an investigation into the relationship between Sudden Infant Death Syndrome and environmental temperature. *J R Stat Soc Ser A* 1994; **157**: 191–208.

7 Berger S, Graham N, Zeileis A. Various versatile variances: an object-oriented implementation of clustered covariances in R. *J Stat Softw* 2020; **95**(1): 1–36.

8 Arain M, Campbell MJ, Nicholl JP. Impact of a GP-led walk-in centre on NHS emergency departments. *Emerg Med J* 2014. doi: 10.1136/emermed-2013-202410

9 Framework for Enhanced Reporting of Interrupted Time Series (FERITS). https://www.equator-network.org/library/reporting-guidelines-under-development/reporting-guidelines-under-development-for-observational-studies/#92

10 Ballard M, Olsen HE, Millear A, *et al.* Continuity of community-based healthcare provision during COVID-19: a multicountry interrupted time series analysis. *BMJ Open* 2022; **12**: e052407. doi: 10.1136/bmjopen-2021-052407

Appendix 1

Exponentials and Logarithms

It is simple to understand raising a quantity to a power, so that: $y = x^2$ is equivalent to: $y = x \times x$. This can be generalised to: $y = x^n$ for arbitrary n so $y = x \times x \times \ldots \times x$ n times.

A simple result is that:

$$x^n \times x^m = x^{n+m} \quad \text{(A1.1)}$$

for arbitrary n and m. Thus, for example $3^2 \times 3^4 = 3^6 = 729$. It can be shown that this holds for *any* values of m and n, not just whole numbers.

We define: $x^0 = 1$, because: $x^n = x^{0+n} = x^0 \times x^n = 1 \times x^n$.

A useful extension of the concept of powers is to let n take fractional or negative values. Thus: $y = x^{0.5}$ can be shown to be equivalent to: $y = \sqrt{x}$, because: $x^{0.5} \times x^{0.5} = x^{0.5+0.5} = x^1 = x$ and also: $\sqrt{x} \times \sqrt{x} = x$.

Also: x^{-1} can be shown equivalent to $1/x$, because: $x \times x^{-1} = x^{1-1} = x^0 = 1$.

If $y = x^n$, then the definition of a logarithm of y to the base x is the power that x has to be raised to get y. This is written: $n = log_x(y)$ or "n equals log to the base x of y".

Suppose $y = x^n$ and $z = x^m$. It can be shown from Equation A1.1 that:

$$log_x(y \times z) = n + m = log_x(y) + log_x(z)$$

Thus, when we multiply two numbers we add their logs. This was the basis of the original use of logarithms in that they enabled a transformation whereby arithmetic using multiplications could be done using additions, which are much easier to do by hand. In Appendix 2 we need an equivalent result, namely that:

$$log_x\left(\frac{y}{z}\right) = log_x(y) - log_x(z)$$

In other words, when we log transform the ratio of two numbers we subtract the logs of the two numbers.

The two most common bases are 10, and a strange quantity: e = 2.718..., where the dots indicate that the decimals go on indefinitely. This number e has the useful property that the slope of the curve: $y = e^x$ at any point (x, y) is just y, whereas for all other bases the slope is proportional to y but not exactly equal to it. The formula: $y = e^x$ is often

Statistics at Square Two: Understanding Modern Statistical Application in Medicine, Third Edition.
Michael J. Campbell and Richard M. Jacques.

written: $y = exp(x)$. The logarithms to base e and 10 are often denoted ln and log respectively on calculators, and log and log10 in R. Logs to base e are often called the *natural logarithm*. In this book all logarithms are natural, that is to base e. We can get from one base to the other by noting that: $log_{10}(y) = log_e(y) \times log_{10}(e)$. To find the value of e in R use the fact that: $e^1 = e$, thus:

```
> e<- exp(1)
> e
[1] 2.718282
```

To find $\log_{10}$(e):

```
> log10(e)
[1] 0.4342945
```

Thus: $log_{10}(y) = 0.4343 \times log_e(y)$.
Note, log is just the inverse function to exponential so: $exp(ln(x)) = x$.
For example if x = 23:

```
> exp(log(23))
[1] 23
```

Note, it follows from the definition that for any: $x > 0$, $log_x(1) = 0$.

In this book exponentials and logarithms feature in a number of places. It is much easier to model data as additive terms in a linear predictor and yet often terms, such as risk, behave multiplicatively, as discussed in Chapter 3. Taking logs transforms the model from a

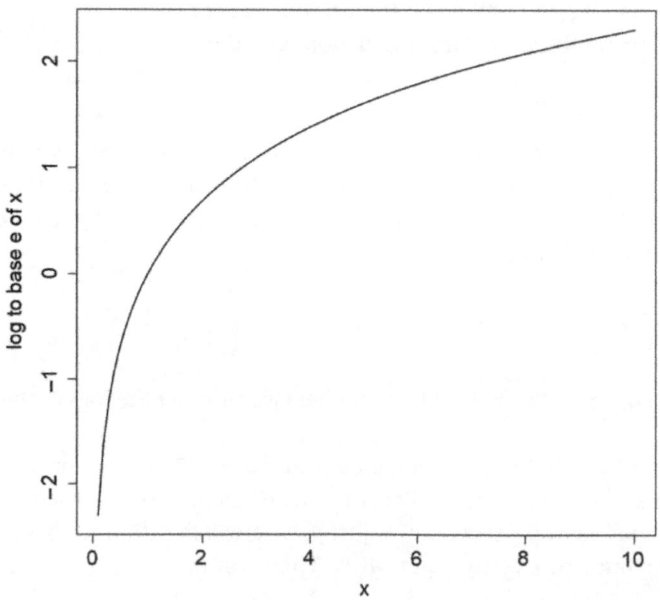

Figure A1.1 $Log_e(x)$ vs x.

multiplicative one to an additive one. Logarithms are also commonly used to transform variables which have a positively skewed distribution, because it has been found that this often makes their distribution closer to a Normal distribution. Many distributions in medicine are positively skewed, such as blood pressure, perhaps because they are effectively truncated at the left hand side but not at the right. Thus, very low blood pressure is rapidly fatal, whereas a high blood pressure takes time to have an effect, so people with very low blood pressure do not appear in samples. Taking logs, of course, will not work if the variable can be 0 or negative and so one cannot take logs of *changes* of variables. A graph of: $log_e(x)$ vs x is shown in Figure A1.1. The line does not plateau, but the rate of increase gets smaller as x increases.

Appendix 2

Maximum Likelihood and Significance Tests

Summary

This appendix gives a brief introduction to the use of *maximum likelihood*, which was the method used to fit the models in the earlier chapters. We describe the *Wald test* and the *likelihood ratio (LR) test* and link the latter to the *deviance*. Further details are given in Clayton and Hills.[1]

A2.1 Binomial Models and Likelihood

A *model* is a structure for describing data and consists of two parts. The first part describes how the explanatory variables are combined in a linear fashion to give a linear predictor. This is then transformed by a function known as a *link* function to give predicted or fitted values of the outcome variable for an individual. The second part of the model describes the probability distribution of the outcome variable about the predicted value.

Perhaps the simplest model is the Binomial model. An event happens with a probability π. Suppose the event is the probability of giving birth to a boy and suppose we had five expectant mothers who subsequently gave birth to two boys and three girls. The boys were born to mothers numbered 1 and 3. If π is the probability of a boy the probability of this sequence of events occurring is $\pi \times (1-\pi) \times \pi \times (1-\pi) \times (1-\pi)$. If the mothers had different characteristics, say their age, we might wish to distinguish them and write the probability of a boy for mother i as π_i, and the probability of a girl as $(1 - \pi_i)$ and the probability of the sequence as $\pi_1 \times (1-\pi_2) \times \pi_3 \times (1-\pi_4) \times (1-\pi_5)$. For philosophical and semantic reasons this probability is termed the *likelihood* (in normal parlance likelihood and probability are synonyms) for this particular sequence of events and in this case is written $L(\pi)$. The likelihood is the probability of the data, *given* the model P(D|M).

The process of *maximum likelihood* is to choose values of the πs which maximise the likelihood. In Chapter 3, we discussed models for the πs which are functions of the subject characteristics. For simplicity, here we will consider two extreme cases: (1) the πs are all the same so we have no information to distinguish individuals, (2) each π is determined by the data, and we can choose each π by whether the outcome is a boy or a girl. In the latter

Statistics at Square Two: Understanding Modern Statistical Application in Medicine, Third Edition.
Michael J. Campbell and Richard M. Jacques.

case we can simply choose $\pi_1 = \pi_3 = 1$ and $\pi_2 = \pi_4 = \pi_5 = 0$. This is a *saturated model*, so-called because we saturate the model with parameters, and the maximum number possible is to have as many parameters as there are data points (or strictly *degrees of freedom* (d.f.)). In this case:

$$L(\pi) = 1 \times (1-0) \times 1 \times (1-0) \times (1-0) = 1$$

If the πs are all the same, then $L(\pi) = \pi \times (1-\pi) \times \pi \times (1-\pi) \times (1-\pi) = \pi^2(1-\pi)^3$. In general if there were D boys in N births then $L(\pi) = \pi^D(1-\pi)^{N-D}$. The likelihood, for any particular value of π is a very small number, and it is more convenient to use the natural logarithm (as described in Appendix 1) of the likelihood instead of the likelihood itself. In this way:

$$\log_e[L(\pi)] = D\log_e(\pi) + (N-D)\log_e(1-\pi) \quad \text{(A2.1)}$$

It is simple to show that the value of π that maximises the likelihood is the same value that maximises the log-likelihood.

In the expression A2.1, the data provide N and D and the statistical problem is to see how $\log[L(\pi)]$ varies as we vary π, and to choose the value of π that most closely agrees with the data. This is the value of π that maximises $\log[L(\pi)]$. A graph of the log-likelihood for the data above (two boys and three girls) is given in Figure A2.1.

The maximum occurs at $\pi = 0.4$, which is what one might have guessed. The value at the maximum is given by:

$$\log_e\left[L(\pi_{max})\right] = 2\log_e(0.4) + 3\log_e(1-0.4) = -3.3651$$

The graph, however, is very flat, implying that the maximum is not well estimated. This is because we have very little information with only five observations.

In general, if the sequence of births is not specified the probability of getting D boys out of N births is the binomial probability: $P = \frac{N!}{D!(N-D)!}\pi^D(1-\pi)^{N-D}$ where: $N! = N \times (N-1) \times (N-2) \times \ldots \times 1$. The expression not involving π is only dependent on the data, not the

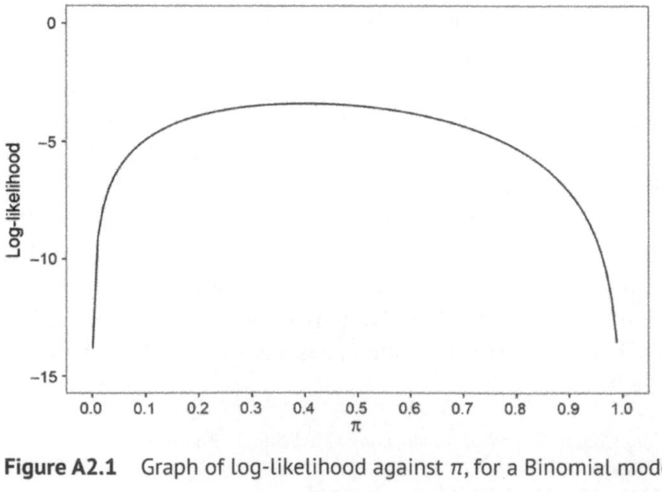

Figure A2.1 Graph of log-likelihood against π, for a Binomial model with $D = 2$ and $N = 5$.

model, and since the data are fixed, it is a constant. The equation for the likelihood is often scaled by the value of the likelihood at the maximum, to give the likelihood ratio, LR(π):

$$LR(\pi) = \frac{L(\pi)}{L(\pi_{max})} \quad 0 < \pi < 1.$$

Thus the constant term is removed. When we take logs this becomes:

$$log_e[LR(\pi)] = log_e[L(\pi)] - log_e[L(\pi_{max})]$$

Again the maximum occurs when $\pi = 0.4$, but in this case the maximum value is 0.

A2.2 The Poisson Model

The Poisson model, discussed in Chapter 6, is useful when the number of subjects N is large and the probability of an event, π, is small. Then the expected number of events $\lambda = N\pi$ is moderate.

In this case the likelihood for an observed count D is $L(\lambda) = e^{-\lambda}\lambda^D$ and the log-likelihood is:

$$\log_e[L(\lambda)] = D\log_e(\lambda) - \lambda.$$

A2.3 The Normal Model

The probability distribution for a variable Y which has a Normal distribution with mean μ and standard deviation σ is given by:

$$\frac{0.3989}{\sigma}\exp\left[\frac{-1}{2}\left(\frac{y-\mu}{\sigma}\right)^2\right]$$

This value changes with differing μ and differing σ. If σ is known (and thus fixed), then this likelihood is simply equal to the above probability but now does not vary with σ and is a function of μ only, which we denote $L(\mu)$.

For a series of observations $y_1, y_2, ..., y_n$ the log-likelihood is:

$$\log_e[L(\mu)] = k - \frac{1}{2\sigma^2}\sum_{i=1}^{n}(y_i - \mu)^2$$

where k is a constant.

A saturated model will have n parameters $\mu_1 = y_1$, $\mu_2 = y_2$, etc. and $\log_e[L(\mu_1, ..., \mu_n)] = k$. Note that this is a constant whatever the model.

Thus the log LR is:

$$\log_e[L(\mu)] = -\frac{1}{2\sigma^2}\sum_{i=1}^{n}(y_i - \mu)^2 \quad \text{(A2.2)}$$

It is easy to show that to *maximise* the log LR we have to minimise the sum on the right-hand side of A2.2, because the quantity on the right is negative and small absolute negative values are bigger than large absolute negative values (−1 is bigger than −2). Thus, we have to choose a value to minimise the sum of squares of the observations from μ. This is the *principle of least squares* described in Chapter 2, and we can see it is equivalent to maximising the likelihood.

The maximum value occurs when:

$$\hat{\mu} = \sum_{i=1}^{n} \frac{y_i}{n} = \bar{y}$$

Suppose we know that adult male height has a Normal distribution. We do not know the mean μ, but we do know the variance to be 15 cm. Imagine ten men selected at random from this population with an average height of 175 cm. The mean of a set of n observations from a Normal distribution with mean μ and variance σ^2 is itself Normally distributed with mean μ and variance σ^2/n.

Then the log LR for these data against a theoretical value μ is:

$$\log_e\left[\mathrm{LR}(\mu)\right] = -\frac{n}{2\sigma^2}(\bar{y} - \mu)^2$$

For our data this is given by:

$$\log_e\left[\mathrm{LR}(\mu)\right] = -\frac{10}{2}\frac{(175 - \mu)^2}{15} \tag{A2.3}$$

This is shown in Figure A2.2 for different values of μ. Curves with this form are called *quadratic*.

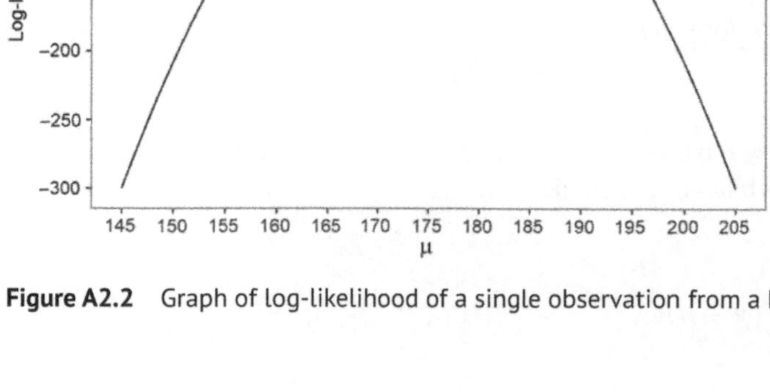

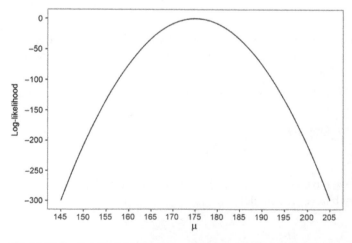

Figure A2.2 Graph of log-likelihood of a single observation from a Normal model.

A2.4 Hypothesis Testing: the Likelihood Ratio Test

Suppose we wished to test the hypothesis that the population from which these men were drawn had a mean height of 170 cm.

Before we can calculate the hypothesis test, we must first use a most useful result for the Normal distribution. The result is that under the Normal distribution the quantity *deviance*, in this case given by:

$$\text{deviance} = -2 \times (\text{observed log LR}) \tag{A2.4}$$

is distributed as a chi-squared distribution. The degrees of freedom depend on the number of extra parameters in the model. In this case there is just one parameter, μ and so there is one degree of freedom.

Our hypothesis is that μ_0 was 170. Then D is $2 \times 10 \times (175 - 170)^2/(2 \times 15) = 16.7$. This is well in excess of the 1% value of a chi-squared distribution with 1 d.f. of 6.63 and so, with our observation of a mean of 175 cm we can reject the null hypothesis that $\mu_0 = 170$.

For non-Normal data the result that $-2 \times$ (observed log LR) is distributed as a chi-squared distribution is approximately true, and the distribution gets closer to a chi-squared distribution as the sample size increases. Returning to our birth data, suppose our null hypothesis was $\pi_0 = 0.5$, that is, boys and girls are equally likely. The log-likelihood is $2 \times \log(0.5) + 3 \times \log(0.5) = -3.4657$ and the corresponding log LR is $-3.4657 - (-3.3651) = -0.1006$.

We have $-2 \times \log \text{LR} = 0.20$, which is much less than the tabulated chi-squared value of 3.84 and so we cannot reject the null hypothesis. Here, the approximation to a chi-squared distribution is likely to be poor because of the small sample size. Intuitively we can see that, because the curve in Figure A2.1 is far from quadratic. However, as the sample size increases it will become closer to a quadratic curve.

The log-likelihood is a measure of *goodness-of-fit* of a model. The greater the log-likelihood the better the fit. Since the absolute value of the log-likelihood is not itself of interest, it is often reported as a log LR compared to some other model. To compare two models many computer programs report the deviance, which in general is minus twice the log LR of two models where one is nested in the other. (Nested means that the model with fewer parameters can be derived from the model with more parameters by setting some of the parameters in the larger model to zero.) Thus: $y = \beta_0 + \beta_1 x$ is nested in $y = \beta_0 + \beta_1 x + \beta_2 x^2$)

Any model is nested within a saturated model which includes the maximum number of terms in the model (say as many terms as there are observations), so the deviance of a model against the saturated model gives an overall goodness-of-fit of the model. For the birth data above, the saturated model had five parameters, the likelihood was 1 and the log-likelihood 0, and so the deviance in this case is the same as the log-likelihood times minus two. The deviance has d.f. equal to the difference between the number of parameters in the model and the number of parameters in the saturated model.

The deviance is really a measure of badness-of-fit, not goodness-of-fit; a large deviance indicates a bad fit. If one model is nested within another, then they can be compared using the differences in their deviances. The change in deviance is minus twice the log

LR for the two models because the log-likelihood for the saturated model occurs in both deviances and cancels. The d.f. for this test are found by subtracting the d.f. for the two deviances.

A2.5 The Wald Test

When the data are not Normally distributed, the shape of the log LR is no longer quadratic. However, as can be seen from Figure A2.1, it is often approximately so, especially for large samples and there can be advantages in terms of simplicity to using the best quadratic approximation rather than the true likelihood.

Consider a likelihood for a parameter θ of a probability model and let M be the most likely value of θ. A simple quadratic expression is:

$$\log\left[LR(\theta)\right]=-\frac{1}{2}\left(\frac{M-\theta}{S}\right)^2$$

This is known as the Wald LR and has a maximum value of 0 when $M=\theta$; it can be used to approximate the true log LR. The parameter S is known as the standard error (SE) of the estimate and is used to scale the curve. Small values give sharp peaks of the quadratic curve and large values give flatter peaks. S is chosen to give the closest approximation to the true likelihood *in the region of its most likely value.*

For the binary data given above, with D events out of N the values of M and S are:

$$M=\frac{D}{N}, \text{ and } S=\sqrt{\frac{M(1-M)}{N}}$$

For $D = 2$ and $N = 5$ we get $M = 0.4$ and $S = 0.22$.

Under the null hypothesis of $\theta = 0.5$, we find that for the Wald LR $-2 \times \log_e$ LR is:

$$\left(\frac{0.4-0.5}{0.22}\right)^2=0.21$$

This is close to the log LR value of 0.20 and once again is not statistically significant. This test is commonly used because computer programs obligingly produce estimates of SEs of parameters. This is equivalent to the z-test described in *Statistics at Square One* of b/SE(b).

A2.6 The Score Test

The score test features less often and so we will not describe it in detail. It is based on the gradient of the log LR curve at the null hypothesis. The gradient is often denoted by U and known as the score, evaluated at the null value of the parameter θ_0. Since the slope of a curve at its maximum is 0, if the null hypothesis coincides with the most likely value, then clearly $U = 0$. The score test is based on the fact that under the null hypothesis U^2/V is approximately distributed as a chi-squared distribution with 1 d.f., where V is an estimate of the square of the SE of the score.

A2.7 Which Method to Choose?

For non-Normal data, the methods given above are all approximations. The advantage of the log LR method is that it gives the same *p*-value even if the parameter is transformed (such as by taking logarithms), and so is the generally preferred method. If the three methods give seriously different results, it means that the quadratic approximations are not sufficiently close to the true log-likelihood curve in the region going from the null value to the most likely value. This is particularly true if the null value and the most likely value are very far apart, and in this case the choice of the statistical method is most unlikely to affect our scientific conclusions. The Wald test can be improved by a suitable transformation. For example, in a model which includes an odds ratio (OR), reformulating the model for a log OR will improve the quadratic approximation, which is another reason why the log OR is a suitable model in Chapter 3.

All three methods can be generalised to test a number of parameters simultaneously. However, if one uses a computer program to fit two models, one of which is a subset of the other, then the log-likelihood or the deviance is usually given for each model from which one can derive the log LR for the two models. If the larger model contains two or more parameters more than the smaller model, then the log LR test of whether the enhanced model significantly improves the fit of the data is a test of all the extra parameters simultaneously.

The parameter estimates and their SEs are given for each term in a model in a computer output, from which the Wald tests can be derived for each parameter. Thus, the simple Wald test tests each parameter separately, not simultaneously with the others. Examples are given in the relevant chapters.

A2.8 Confidence Intervals

The conventional approach to confidence intervals (CIs) is to use the Wald approach. Thus, an approximate 95% CI of a population parameter, for which we have an estimate and the SE is given by an estimate minus 2 × SE to estimate plus 2 × SE. Thus for the birth data an approximate 95% CI is given by $0.6 - 2 \times 0.22$ to $0.6 + 2 \times 0.22 = 0.16$ to 1.04. This immediately shows how poor the approximation is because we cannot have a proportion > 1. (for better approximations see Altman *et al.*).[2] As in the case of the Wald test, the approximation is improved by a suitable transformation, which is why in Chapter 3 we worked on the log OR, rather than the OR itself. However, it is possible to calculate CIs directly from the likelihood, which do not require a transformation, and these are occasionally given in the literature. These are known as *profile* based confidence intervals For further details see Clayton and Hills.[1]

A2.9 Deviance Residuals for Binary Data

Suppose we have observed binary data $y_i = 0$ or 1 on N subjects and fitted data $\hat{y}_i$. Thus: $D = \Sigma y_i$, $ni = 1$ for all I and $N = \Sigma n_i$. The deviance residuals for binary data are defined as:

$$d_i = \sqrt{2\left[y_i \log\left(\frac{y_i}{\hat{y}_i}\right) + (n_i - y_i)\log\left(\frac{n_i - y_i}{n_i - \hat{y}_i}\right)\right]} \quad (A.2.5)$$

This part in square brackets is effectively the ratio of the log likelihood of the observed data for data point i and the null log likelihood for data point i.

If we square these and sum them over i we get the deviance, and each d_i is the individual contribution of i to the deviance.

A2.10 Example: Derivation of the Deviances and Deviance Residuals Given in Table 3.3

A2.10.1 Grouped Data

From Table 3.2 for the whole group we have $D = 32$ and $N = 263$ and so under the null hypothesis the best estimate of the probability of dying after six months of follow-up for the whole group is $\pi. = 32/263 = 0.1217$. From Equation A2.1 we have:

$\log[L(\pi)] = 32 \ln(0.1217) + 231 \ln(1 - 0.1217) = -97.374$ with 262 degrees of freedom.

Under the alternative hypothesis we have: $D_0 = 21$, $N_0 = 131$. $\pi_0 = 0.160$ and $D_1 = 11$, $N_1 = 132$ and $\pi_1 = 0.083$ and so:

$\log[L(\pi)] = 21 \times \ln(0.1603) + 110 \times \ln(1 - 0.1603) + 11\ln(0.0833) + 121 \times \ln(1 - 0.0833) = -95.525$ with 261 degrees of freedom. Thus the null deviance is $-2[-97.374 + 95.525] = 3.698$ with $262 = 261 = 1$ degree of freedom as shown in Table 3.3.

There are two null deviance residuals, one for the treatment group and one for the control. For each we find the observed log likelihood ratio (LLR) and then get the deviance residual by deviance residual = sign (Obs - Fit) × √(2 × LLR) Thus: $d_0 = \sqrt{2} \times [21 \times \log(0.1603/0.1217) + 110 \times \log(1 - 0.1603)/(1 - 0.1217)] = 1.297$ and since $0.1603 - 0.1217$ is positive we get $d_0 = 1.297$.

Also $d_1 = \sqrt{2} \times (11 \times \log(0.0833/0.1217) + 121 \times \log(1 - 0.0833)/(1 - 0.1217)) = 1.419$ and since $0.0833 - 0.1217$ is negative we get $d_1 = -1.419$.

For the alternative hypothesis, the model fits perfectly so the deviance residuals are zero.

A2.10.2 Ungrouped Data

Under the null hypothesis, there are two residuals, for $y_i = 0$ or 1.

From Equation A2.5 when $y_i = 0$ we have: $d_i = \sqrt{2 \times \log\left(\frac{1}{1-\hat{y}}\right)}$ and when $y_i = 1$:

$d_i = \sqrt{2 \times \log\left(\frac{1}{\hat{y}}\right)}$. Since $\hat{y} = 0.1217$ we get $d_i = -0.509$ or 2.052 respectively.

Under the alternative hypothesis, there are four residuals: for treatment and when $y_i = 0$ or 1 and for control when $y_i = 0$ or 1.

The values of $\hat{y}$ under treatment and control are 0.0833 and 0.1603 respectively and this leads to residuals of −0.417 and 2.229 for treatment and −0.591 and 1.913 for control as given in Table 3.3

References

1 Clayton D, Hills M. *Statistical Models in Epidemiology*. Oxford: OUP, 1993.

2 Altman DG, Machin D, Bryant TN, Gardner MJ, eds. *Statistics with Confidence*, 2nd edn. London: BMJ Books, 2000.

Appendix 3

Bootstrapping and Variance Robust Standard Errors

A3.1 The Bootstrap

Bootstrapping is a computer intensive method for estimating parameters and confidence intervals (CIs) for models that requires fewer assumptions about the distribution of the data than parametric methods. It is becoming much easier to carry out and is available on most modern computer packages.

All the models so far discussed require assumptions concerning the sampling distribution of the estimate of interest. If the sample size is large and we wish to estimate a CI for a mean, then the underlying population distribution is not important because the central limit theorem will ensure that the sampling distribution is approximately Normal. However, if the sample size is small we can only assume a t-distribution if the underlying population distribution can be assumed Normal. If this is not the case then the interval cannot be expected to cover the population value with the specified confidence. However, we have information on the distribution of the population from the distribution of the sample data. So-called "bootstrap" estimates (from the expression "pulling oneself up by one's bootstraps") utilise this information, by making repeated random samples of the same size as the original sample from the data, with replacement using a computer. Suitable references are Efron and Tibshirani,[1] Chernick and LaBudde[2] and Bland and Altman.[3]

We seek to mimic in an appropriate manner the way the sample is collected from the population in the bootstrap samples from the observed data. The "with replacement" means that any observation can be sampled more than once. It is important because sampling without replacement would simply give a random permutation of the original data, with many statistics such as the mean being exactly the same. It turns out that "with replacement" is the best way to do this if the observations are independent; if they are not then other methods, beyond the scope of this book, are needed. The standard error (SE) or CI is estimated from the variability of the statistic derived from the bootstrap samples. The point about the bootstrap is that it produces a variety of values, whose variability reflects the SE which would be obtained if samples were repeatedly taken from the whole population.

Suppose we wish to calculate a 95% CI for a mean. We take a random sample of the data, of the same size as the original sample, and calculate the mean of the data in this random sample. We do this repeatedly, say 999 times. We now have 999 means. If these are ordered

Statistics at Square Two: Understanding Modern Statistical Application in Medicine, Third Edition.
Michael J. Campbell and Richard M. Jacques.

in increasing value a bootstrap 95% CI for the mean would be from the 25th to the 975th values. This is known as the *percentile method* and although it is an obvious choice, it is not the best method of bootstrapping because it can have a bias, which one can estimate and correct for. This leads to methods, such as the *bias-corrected method* and the *bias-corrected and accelerated (BCa) method*, the latter being the preferred option. When analysis involves an explicit model we can use the "parametric bootstrap". In this case, the model is fitted and the estimated coefficients, the fitted values and residuals stored. The residuals are then randomly sampled with replacement and then these bootstrapped residuals are added to the fitted values to give a new dependent variable. The model is then estimated again and the procedure repeated. The sequence of estimated coefficients gives us the distribution from which we can derive the bootstrap statistics.

Using these methods, valid bootstrap CIs can be constructed for all common estimators, such as a proportion, a median, or a difference in means, and valid p-values for hypothesis tests, provided the data are independent and come from the same population.

The number of samples required depends on the type of estimator: 50–200 are adequate for a CI for a mean, but 1000 are required for a CI of, say, the 2.5% or 97.5% centiles.

A3.2 Example of the Bootstrap

Consider the beta-endorphin concentrations from 11 runners described by Dale *et al.*[4] and also described in Altman *et al.* (Chapter 13)[5] given in Table A3.1. To calculate a 95% CI for the median using a bootstrap we proceed as follows:

Table A3.1 Calculating a bootstrap confidence interval for a median.

	Beta-endorphin concentrations in pmol/l	**Median**
Original sample:	66, 71.2, 83.0, 83.6, 101, 107.6, 122, 143, 160, 177, 414	107.6
Bootstrap 1:	143, 107.6, 414, 160, 101, 177, 107.6, 160, 160, 160, 101	160
Bootstrap 2:	122, 414, 101, 83.6, 143, 107.6, 101, 143, 143, 143, 107.6	122
Bootstrap 3:	122, 414, 160, 177, 101, 107.6, 83.6, 177, 177, 107.6, 107.6	122
etc. 999 times		

The medians are then ordered by increasing value. The 25th and the 975th values out of 1000 give the percentile estimates of the 95% CI. Using 999 replications we find that the BCa method gives a 95% bootstrap CI 71.2 to 143.0 pmol/l. This contrasts with 71.2 to 177 pmol/l using standard methods given in Chapter 5 of Altman *et al.*[5] This suggests that the lower limit for the standard method is probably about right but the upper limit may be too high.

When the standard and the bootstrap methods agree, we can be more confident about the inference we are making and this is an important use of the bootstrap. When they disagree more caution is needed, but the relatively simple assumptions required by the bootstrap method for validity mean that in general it is to be preferred.

It may seem that the best estimator of the median for the population is the median of the bootstrap estimates, but this turns out not to be the case and one should quote the sample median as the best estimate of the population median.

The main advantage of the bootstrap is that it frees the investigator from making inappropriate assumptions about the distribution of an estimator in order to make inferences. A particular advantage is that it is available when the formula cannot be derived and it may provide better estimates when the formulae are only approximate.

The so-called "naive" bootstrap makes the assumption that the sample is an unbiased simple random sample from the study population. More complex sampling schemes, such as stratified random sampling, may not be reflected by this and more complex bootstrapping schemes may be required. Naive bootstrapping may not be successful in very small samples (say, < 9 observations), which are less likely to be representative of the study population. "In very small samples even a badly fitting parametric analysis may outperform a non-parametric analysis, by providing less variable results at the expense of a tolerable amount of bias."[1]

Perhaps one of the most common uses for bootstrapping in medical research has been for calculating CIs for derived statistics, such as cost-effectiveness ratios, when the theoretical distribution is mathematically difficult. Care is needed for ratios since the denominators in some bootstrap samples can get close to 0, for example when a treatment is not very effective, in which case the cost-effectiveness ratio can approach infinity.

A3.3 Interpreting a Computer Output: The Bootstrap

A3.3.1 Two-sample T-test with Unequal Variances

Suppose we wished to compare deadspace in children with asthma and children without asthma, ignoring other factors, using the data in Table 2.1. A conventional t-test assuming equal variances is given in Table A3.2(i). The difference in means (Asthma – Normal) is −30.125 ml and the conventional CI for this difference is −50.79 to −9.46 ml. However, a simple check, such as graphing the data, shows that the variability between groups is very different, with an s.d. of 7.79 ml for the children with asthma and 25.87 for the children without.

One might wish to see how the CI would be changed using a parametric bootstrap. The output from this procedure is given in Table A3.2(ii), which shows three different bootstrap statistics. The BCa bootstrap CI (the recommended one) is −46.43 to −3.77 ml. This is no longer symmetric about the point estimate and the lower end is closer to 0 than the conventional CI estimate.

A3.4 The Bootstrap in the Medical Literature

Sampaio *et al.*[6] conducted a randomised trial of Internet-delivered cognitive-behavioural therapy for adolescents with irritable bowel syndrome. They randomised 47 adolescents to the treatment and 54 to the control. The outcome was a form of Quality Adjusted Life Year (QALY). For all resources they found the mean difference in QALYs between the two groups as 0.0031 (95% CI 0.0003 to 0.0061) and the mean difference in costs as $184.45. The ratio (the incremental cost effectiveness ratio or ICER) was 59,500. They used a bootstrap method with 5000 samples because the resource costs have a very skewed

Table A3.2 Output illustrating use of the bootstrap to compare two means.

(i) Two-sample t-test with equal variances.

```
    Two Sample t-test

data:  a1 and a2
t = -3.1493, df = 13, p-value = 0.007682
alternative hypothesis: true difference in means is not equal to 0
95 percent confidence interval:
 -50.790317  -9.459683
sample estimates:
mean of  x mean of y
    52.875    83.000

Difference in means -30.125
Standard deviations with and without asthma 7.790791 25.87148
```

(ii) Bootstrap confidence interval.

```
Bootstrap confidence interval calculations
Based on 1000 bootstrap replicates

Intervals :
Level      Normal              Percentile            BCa
95%   (-50.08, -10.01 )    (-48.85,   -8.82 )   (-46.43,   -3.77 )
```

distribution. The authors did not state which bootstrap method they used but did state the software (Stata). They bootstrapped sampled the pairs (costs, QALYS) and found the proportion of pairs whose ratio was greater than $80,000 was 71%, that is, if the provider was willing to pay $80,000 there was a 71% chance of the treatment being cost effective. This is an interesting example of authors making a statement about the probability of a treatment working, which is essentially a Bayesian statement (see Appendix 4), without using pre-specified prior distributions, but instead using the empirical distributions provided by the bootstrap sample.

A3.5 Robust or Sandwich Estimate SEs

The robust or sandwich estimate SE is now a common feature in analyses and is incorporated in many packages. It was first described by Huber[7] and later by White.[8] The terminology is somewhat controversial. It is "robust" in the sense that *if* the model is the one we describe, *except* that the variance is not constant as is normally assumed, *then* the SEs given by the procedure reflect better what we understand by SEs under repeated sampling than those given by the standard model. It is not "robust" in the sense of a non-parametric test, where we can drop a Normality assumption, or if our model for the predictor variable is actually wrong (e.g. if the relationship is not actually linear). It is called the "sandwich" estimator because in matrix notation the estimate brackets are either side of a correction factor, thus two pieces of bread with a filling.

Recall that the least squares estimate of β for the model $y_i = \alpha + \beta x_i + \varepsilon_i$ is:

$$b = \frac{\sum_{i=1}^{n}(y_i - \bar{y})(x_i - \bar{x})}{\sum_{i=1}^{n}(x_i - \bar{x})^2}$$

Also recall that for any constants a and b and random variable X, $Var(aX - b) = a^2 Var(X)$. Thus:

$$\text{Var}(b) = \frac{\sum_{i=1}^{n} Var(y_i)(x_i - \bar{x})^2}{\left[\sum_{i=1}^{n}(x_i - \bar{x})^2\right]^2}$$

Conventionally, we assume: $Var(y_i) = \sigma^2$, and so the term: $\sum_{i=1}^{n}(x_i - \bar{x})^2$ cancels and we get the usual least squares estimate. However, suppose we were unwilling to assume a constant variance and instead had: $Var(y_i) = \sigma_i^2$. We need an estimate of σ_i^2 and one suggestion is to use the square of the residual e_i. Since σ^2 is usually estimated by: $\sum_{i=1}^{n} e_i^2 / (n - p)$ where p is the number of parameters in the model, we would need to multiply the estimate by $n/(n-p)$ to allow for the fact that a and b are estimates (p = 2 in this case). At first sight one is estimating n + p parameters (the n residuals and the p regression coefficients) with only n data points. However, usually there are constraints, such as we assume for a two sample t-test the variances are constant within groups and so the robust SEs are based on a number of degrees of freedom. In any case, because the variance is not the main focus of the analysis this procedure turns out to give reasonable estimates. A plot e_i^2 against: $(x_i - \bar{x})^2$ will indicate whether a robust estimate will give markedly different results: a positive slope shows that the variance of the residual increases with x, and the robust SE will be bigger than the conventional estimate, a negative slope will indicate the opposite.

There have been many suggestions of methods to allow for small sample bias and leverage (see Chapter 2 for a discussion of leverage). These are described in Mansournia *et al.*[9]

Robust SEs have also been extended to estimate the SEs of parameters of non-linear models such as logistic regression, but here they are only an approximation and should be used with more caution.

A3.6 Interpreting a Computer Output: Robust SEs for Unequal Variances

Consider again the comparison of deadspace in children with asthma and children without asthma. As discussed in *Statistics at Square One* (p. 126), if one is in doubt about the equal variance assumption, rather than use a pooled variance estimate, one can combine the variances for each mean to get: $\frac{s_1^2}{n_1}+\frac{s_2^2}{n_2}$ and adjust the d.f. using either Welch's or Satterthwaite's approximation. This is shown in Table A3.3(i). Note that the *p*-value of 0.021 is much larger than the 0.0077 obtained assuming equal variances given in Table A3.2. One can obtain the same estimate of the SE using robust regression (Table A3.3(ii)), with various robust SE options (HC0, HC2 and HC3). The HC2 option corresponds to the Welch test, and the HC3 option is often recommended since it is the most conservative. Note, however, that to find the *p*-value and CI, with small sample sizes such as we have here, we have to use the Satterthwaite adjustment of the degrees of freedom given in *Statistics at Square One* (p. 125).

The main advantage of robust regression is that it fits seamlessly into a regression framework, and so can be used when the number of explanatory variables is more than one. In some packages there is an option to use robust SEs. As with the unequal variance *t*-test, it is less powerful than conventional methods if the assumptions for the model are met, but is better if there is significant heterogeneity of variance. For large samples the loss of efficiency is slight.

A comparison of the CIs given by the different methods is given in Table A3.4

Note that, in contrast to the bootstrap estimate, the other Cls are symmetric about the estimate. This is because the robust SE can cope with variance heterogeneity, but not with skewness, which these data also display. The robust CIs are all wider than the one that assumes equal variance.

Table A3.3 Computer output using robust regression for unequal variances.

(i) Two-sample t-test with unequal variances.

```
Welch Two Sample t-test

data:  a1 and a2
t = -2.9653, df = 6.9524, p-value = 0.02111
alternative hypothesis: true difference in means is not equal to 0
95 percent confidence interval:
     -54.180683  -6.069317

sample estimates:
mean of x  mean of y
   52.875     83.000
```

(ii) Regression with robust standard errors: HC0.

```
Coefficient:
             Estimate  Std. Error   t value   Pr(>|t|)
Asthma       -30.1250      9.4126   -3.2005     0.0152

# 95% confidence interval
                   2.5 %       97.5 %
Asthma         -52.41328    -7.836718
```

(Continued)

Table A3.3 (Continued)

(iii) Regression with robust standard errors: HC2.

```
Coefficient:
                Estimate     Std. Error     t value    Pr(>|t|)
Asthma          -30.1250        10.1590     -2.9653     0.02111

# 95% confidence interval
                  2.5 %       97.5 %
Asthma      -54.18068   -6.069317
```

(iv) Regression with robust standard errors: HC3.

```
Coefficient:

            Estimate  Std. Error  t value      Pr(>|t|)
Asthma       -30.125      10.965  -2.7474     0.0288025

# 95% confidence interval
                    2.5 %       97.5 %
Asthma        -56.08861   -4.161391
```

Table A3.4 Comparison of confidence intervals for a difference in means by various methods.

Method	**Estimate 95%CI**
Equal variance t-test	−50.79 to −9.46
Welch test	−54.18 to −6.07
Robust HC0	−52.41 to −7.84
Robust HC2	−54.18 to −6.07
Robust HC3	−56.09 to −4.16
Bootstrap BCA	−46.43 to −3.77

A3.7 Other Uses of Robust Regression

- When data are clustered, it is reasonable to assume the variances are the same within clusters, but the data within clusters are correlated (see Chapter 5).
- To get valid estimates for the SEs of relative risks (see Chapter 6).

These are described further in Mansournia *et al.*[9]

A3.8 Reporting the Bootstrap and Robust SEs in the Literature

- State the method of bootstrap used, such as percentile or bias corrected.
- State the number of replications for the bootstrap.

- State what type of robust SE was used.
- Always check assumptions and compare the robust SEs with the usual output to see how deviations can affect the results.

A3.9 Frequently Asked Question

What are the Different Meanings of "Robust" in Statistics?

There are a number of uses of the term "robust" in statistics. The median is described as a robust measure of location since its value is not affected by outlying points. The bootstrap is robust because it does not require the assumption of Normality. Robust SEs are robust against heterogeneous measures of variability. The t-test is said to be robust against departures from Normality. Alas there is no such thing as a free lunch, and one buys validity at the cost of accuracy. The more assumptions one is willing to make about how a set of data is generated (and these assumptions are true) then the more precise one can be.

References

1 Efron B, Tibshirani RJ. *An Introduction to the Bootstrap*. New York: Chapman and Hall, 1993.

2 Chernick MR, LaBudde RA. *An Introduction to Bootstrap methods with Applications to R*. Hoboken, NJ: Wiley Applied Probability and Statistics, 2014.

3 Bland JM, Altman DG. Statistics notes: bootstrap resampling methods. *BMJ* 2015; **350**: h2622.

4 Dale G, Fleetwood JA, Weddell A, Elllis RD, Sainsbury JRC. β-endorphin: a factor in "fun-run" collapse. *BrMed J* 1987; **294**: 1004.

5 Altman DG, Machin D, Bryant TN, Gardner MJ, eds. *Statistics with Confidence*, 2nd edn. London: BMJ Books, 2000.

6 Sampaio F, Bonnert M, Olén O, *et al.* Cost-effectiveness of internet-delivered cognitive-behavioural therapy for adolescents with irritable bowel syndrome. *BMJ Open* 2019; **9**: e023881. doi: 10.1136/bmjopen-2018-023881

7 Huber PJ. The behaviour of maximum likelihood estimates under non-standard conditions. In: *Proceedings of the Fifth Berkeley Symposium on Mathematical Statistics and Probability*, Vol. **1**. Eds. LM Le Cam and J Neyman. Berkeley, CA: University of California Press, 1967, 221–33.

8 White H. A heteroskedasticity-consistent covariance matrix estimator and a direct test for heteroskedasticity. *Econometrika* 1980; **48**: 817–30.

9 Mansournia MA, Nazemipour M, Naimi AI, Collins GS, Campbell MJ. Reflections on modern methods: demystifying robust standard errors for epidemiologists. *Inte J Epidemiol* 2021; **50**(1): 346–51. doi: 10.1093/ije/dyaa260

Appendix 4

Bayesian Methods

Consider two clinical trials of equal size for the treatment of headache. One is a known analgesic against placebo, and the other is a homoeopathic treatment against placebo. Both give identical *p*-values (< 0.05). Which would you believe? The traditional frequentist approach described in the book does not enable one formally to incorporate beliefs about the efficacy of treatment that one might have held before the experiment, but this can be done using *Bayesian methods*.[1]

Bayes' theorem appeared in a posthumous publication in 1763 by Thomas Bayes, a non-conformist minister from Tunbridge Wells. It gives a simple and uncontroversial result in probability theory, relating probabilities of events before an experiment (*a priori*) to probabilities of events after an experiment (*a posteriori*). The link between the prior and the posterior is the *likelihood*, described in Appendix 2. Specific uses of the theorem have been the subject of considerable controversy for many years and it is only in recent years that a more balanced and pragmatic perspective has emerged.[2] An excellent primer on applications of Bayesian methods to health outcomes is freely available from the Centre for Health Economics and Bayesian Statistics (CHEBS) in Sheffield.[3] A useful review for clinicians has been given by Ferreira *et al.*[4]

A4.1 Bayes' Theorem

Very roughly, the risk to a mother of having a baby with Down's syndrome is 1 in 1000 if she is aged under 40, and 1 in 100 if she is 40 or above.[5] Using the notation P(D|age) to indicate the probability of having a baby with Down's given one's age, we have $P(D|age < 40) = 0.001$ and $P(D|age \geq 40) = 0.01$. If one saw a baby with Down's what is the chance the mother is less than 40? What we want is $P(age < 40|D)$. Bayes' Theorem allows us to find this value:

$$P(\text{age} < 40 \mid D) = P(D \mid \text{age} < 40) \times P(\text{age} < 40) / P(D)$$

$P(age < 40)$ is the probability that a mother is less than 40, and P(D) is the overall probability of a mother having a Down's syndrome baby. Given only two age groups:

Statistics at Square Two: Understanding Modern Statistical Application in Medicine, Third Edition.
Michael J. Campbell and Richard M. Jacques.

$$P(D) = P(D \mid age < 40)P(age < 40) + P(D \mid age \geq 40)P(age \geq 40)$$

In the UK about 5% of mothers are aged ≥ 40 when they give birth so:

$$P(D) = 0.001 \times 0.95 + 0.01 \times 0.05 = 0.00145$$

Thus P(age < 40|D) = 0.001 × 0.95/0.00145 = 0.66. Thus, the chances that a baby with Down's syndrome has a mother aged < 40 is greater than 50%. This slightly surprising result is due to the fact that most babies have young mothers.

Another situation to which Bayes' theorem can be applied is diagnostic testing; a doctor's prior belief about whether a patient has a particular disease (based on knowledge of the prevalence of the disease in the community and the patient's symptoms) will be modified by the result of the test. In this case Bayes' theorem can be written as:[6]

Odds of disease given a positive test = odds of disease before the test × LR+

Where LR+ is the likelihood ratio for a positive test and is:

$$LR+ = \frac{Probability\ of\ +ve\ test\ with\ disease}{Probability\ of\ +ve\ test\ without\ disease}$$

In general, given a parameter θ which we want to make inferences about and given some data y, Bayes' Theorem states:

$$P(\theta \mid y) = \frac{P(y \mid \theta) \times P(\theta)}{P(y)}$$

Here p(θ) is the prior distribution of θ. It doesn't necessarily imply time, but rather summarises what we know about θ, either from subjective beliefs, earlier studies or a combination of the two. When y is continuous, the evaluation of P(y) involves integrating over all possible values of y and this can be computationally challenging.

Instead of confidence intervals (CI), we have prediction intervals which is what one would like a CI to be: "a range of values within which one is 95% certain with a given probability that the true value of a parameter really lies". Under certain circumstances, 95% CIs calculated in the conventional (frequentist) manner can be interpreted in this way.[7]

A4.2 Uses of Bayesian Methods

Bayesian methods enable one to make statements such as: "the probability that you have a disease given a positive test result is 0.99" or: "the probability that the new treatment is better than the old is 0.95". It can be argued that a Bayesian approach allows results to be presented in a form that is most suitable for decisions. Bayesian methods interpret data from a study in the light of external evidence and judgement, and the form in which conclusions are drawn contributes naturally to decision-making.[8] Prior plausibility of hypotheses is taken into account, just as when interpreting the results of a diagnostic test. Scepticism about large treatment effects can be formally expressed and used in cautious interpretation of results that cause surprise. Procedures which specify prior distributions for all the parameters in a model are known as "fully Bayesian".

One of the main difficulties with Bayesian methods is the choice of the prior distribution. Different analysts may choose different priors, and so the same data set analysed by different investigators could lead to different conclusions. A commonly chosen prior is an *uninformative prior*, which assigns equal probability to all values over the possible range and leads to analyses that are possibly less subjective than analyses that use priors based on, say, clinical judgement. However what is uninformative on one scale is not necessarily uninformative on a different scale. For example, if the random variable X has a uniform distribution of the line 0 to 1, the random variable X^2 does not and so sensitivity analyses on these so-called "vague" priors should be undertaken.

Empirical Bayes methods are procedures for statistical inference in which the prior distribution is estimated from the data. This compares to standard Bayesian methods, for which the prior distribution is fixed before any data are observed. Empirical Bayes may be viewed as an approximation to a fully Bayesian treatment of a hierarchical model wherein the parameters at the highest level of the hierarchy are set to their most likely values instead of being integrated out. Empirical Bayes' methods lead to *shrinkage estimators*. These are similar to the ideas in meta-analysis whereby estimates from small samples are "shrunk" toward an overall mean more than estimates from large samples. It is particularly useful in spatial mapping, whereby estimates in one area of a country use information about contiguous areas.[9] A recent e-book explaining empirical Bayes is available here: https://drob.gumroad.com/l/empirical-bayes

There are philosophical differences between Bayesians and frequentists, such as the nature of probability, but these should not interfere with a sensible interpretation of data. A Bayesian perspective leads to an approach to clinical trials that is claimed to be more flexible and ethical than traditional methods.[2] Bayesian methods do not supplant traditional methods, but complement them. In this book the area of greatest overlap would be in random effects models, described in Chapter 5 and meta-analysis in Chapter 7. Time series methods, such as interrupted time series described in Chapter 8, which accumulate prior data to make future predictions, are also suitable to Bayesian methods.

A4.3 Computing in Bayes

The main tool in Bayesian computation is a simulation technique Markov chain Monte Carlo (MCMC). The idea of MCMC is in a sense to bypass the mathematical operations rather than to implement them. Bayesian inference is solved by randomly drawing a very large simulated sample from the posterior distribution. The point is that if we have a sufficiently large sample from any distribution then we effectively have that whole distribution in front of us. Anything we want to know about the distribution we can calculate from the sample. This is implemented in a package called Winbugs, but Bayesian methods are in the package Stan (https://mc-stan.org) and are also now available in R.[10]

A4.4 Reading and Reporting Bayesian Methods in the Literature

A checklist for clinicians for reading papers using Bayesian statistics has been given.[11] The checklist was designed to help clinicians interpret the results of a phase III randomised clinical trial analysed by Bayesian methods, even clinicians with no particular knowledge of statistics.

Three items were considered essential to report: specification of the prior, source of the prior (when prior is informative) and the effect size point estimate with its credible interval.

- Report the pre-experiment probabilities and specify how they were determined. In most practical situations, the particular form of the prior information has little influence on the final outcome because it is overwhelmed by the weight of experimental evidence.
- Report the post-trial probabilities and their intervals. Often the mode of the posterior distribution is reported, with the 2.5 and 97.5 centiles (the 95% prediction interval). It can be helpful to plot the posterior distribution.

A4.5 Reading about the Results of Bayesian Methods in the Medical Literature

Thorpe *et al.*[12] looked at the effect of police cameras on the number and severity of casualties at 46 mobile camera sites in an area of the UK. They contrasted empirical Bayes methods with fully Bayes methods. They used data before the installation of the cameras to build an empirical distribution for prediction of casualties after the introduction of cameras. They argued that empirical Bayes methods only produce point estimates and that it is better to have a proper posterior distribution. They stated that using empirical Bayes, one would have estimated 21 casualties were prevented, but using full Bayes they were able to get a posterior distribution and found the median estimate of only 8 casualties were prevented by the cameras. For some reason they did not attach credible intervals to these estimates, but they did give a range of costs saved of £12,500–15,000 per annum.

References

1 Bland JM, Altman DG. Bayesians and frequentists. *BMJ* 1998; **317**: 1151–52.

2 Spiegelhalter DJ, Abrams KR, Myles IP. *Bayesian Approaches to Clinical Trials and Health-care Evaluation*. Chichester: John Wiley, 2004.

3 O'Hagan A, Luce BR. *A Primer on Bayesian Statistics in Health Economic and Outcomes Research*, 2004. http://gemini-grp.com/Bayes/OHaganPrimer.pdf

4 Ferreira D, Barthoulot M, Pottecher J, Torp KD, Diemunsch P, Meyer N. Theory and practical use of Bayesian methods in interpreting clinical trial data: a narrative review. *British Journal of Anaesthesia* 2020; **125**(2): 201–07.

5 Downs syndrome risk by age. https://www.newhealthadvisor.org/down-syndrome-risk-by-age.htm.

6 Campbell MJ. *Statistics at Square One*, 12th edn. Hoboken, NJ: Wiley-Blackwell, 2021. Chapter 5.

7 Burton PR, Gurrin LC, Campbell MJ. Clinical significance not statistical significance: a simple Bayesian alternative to *P*-values. *J Epidemiol Commun Health* 1998; **52**: 318–23.

8 Lilford RJ, Braunholtz D. The statistical basis of public policy a paradigm shift is overdue. *BMJ* 1996; **313**: 603–07.

9 Lawson AB. *Bayesian Disease Mapping: Hierarchical Modeling in Spatial Epidemiology*. Boca Raton, Florida: CRC Press, 2013.

10 Johnson AA, Ott MQ, Dogucu M. *Bayes Rules! An Introduction to Applied Bayesian Modeling*. CRC Press, 2022.

11 Ferreira D, Barthoulot M, Pottecher J, Torp KD, Diemunsch P, Meyer N. A consensus checklist to help clinicians interpret clinical trial results analysed by Bayesian methods. *British Journal of Anaesthesia* 2020; **125**(2): 208–15.

12 Thorpe N, Fawcett L. Linking road casualty and clinical data to assess the effectiveness of mobile safety enforcement cameras: a before and after study. *BMJ Open* 2012; **2**: e001304. doi:10.1136/bmjopen-2012-001304

Appendix 5

R codes

A5.1 R Code for Chapter 2

R libraries

Plots are drawn using the ggplot[1] library and the moderndive[2] library is used to add the lines with parallel slopes in Figure 2.2.

```
library(ggplot2)
library(moderndive)
```

Table 2.1 Lung function data on 15 children.

```
# Create a data frame of the lung function data

Lung.Function <-
    data.frame(Child.Number = c(1:15),
      Deadspace = c(44,31,43,45,56,79,57,56,58,92,78,64,88,112,101),
      Height = c(110,116,124,129,131,138,142,150,153,155,156,159,164,168,174),
      Asthma = c(1,0,1,1,1,0,1,1,1,0,0,1,0,0,0),
      Age = c(5,5,6,7,7,6,6,8,8,9,7,8,10,11,14),
      Bronchitis = c(0,1,0,0,0,0,0,0,0,1,1,0,1,0,0))

# Create additional variable showing the labels for asthma

Lung.Function$Asthma.Labels <-
    factor(Lung.Function$Asthma,
      labels = c("0" = "Children without asthma", "1" = "Children with asthma"))
```

Statistics at Square Two: Understanding Modern Statistical Application in Medicine, Third Edition.
Michael J. Campbell and Richard M. Jacques.

```
ggplot(data=Lung.Function, aes(x = Height, y = Deadspace))+
    # Add the data points to the plot and set the colour for each group
    geom_point(aes(color = Asthma.Labels, shape = Asthma.Labels), size=2)+
    scale_colour_manual(values = c("Children without asthma"="black", "Children
      with asthma"="darkgrey"))+
    # Add the regression line
    geom_smooth(method="lm",formula = y~x, se=F, colour="black",
      fullrange=T, size=0.5)+
    # Label the x and y axes, setting the limits and breaks
    scale_x_continuous("Height (cm)", limits=c(110,180),
      breaks=seq(110,180,10))+
    scale_y_continuous("Deadspace (ml)", limits=c(29,120),
      breaks=seq(30,120,10))+
    # Use the black and white theme with size 10 font
    theme_bw(base_size=10)+
    # Set the legend title, background and position
    theme(legend.title = element_blank(), legend.background = element_blank(),
      legend.position = c(0.15,0.9))+
    # Remove the major and minor grid lines
    theme(panel.grid.major = element_blank(), panel.grid.minor = element_blank())
```

Figure 2.1 Deadspace versus height, ignoring asthma status.

```
ggplot(data=Lung.Function,
      aes(x = Height, y = Deadspace, color = Asthma.Labels, shape =
      Asthma.Labels))+
    # Add the data points to the plot and set the colour for each group
    geom_point(size=2)+
    scale_colour_manual(values = c("Children without asthma"="black", "Children
      with asthma"="darkgrey"))+
    # Add the regression lines
    geom_parallel_slopes(se=F, fullrange=T, size=0.5)+
    # Label the x and y axes, setting the limits and breaks
    scale_x_continuous("Height (cm)", limits=c(110,180),
      breaks=seq(110,180,10))+
    scale_y_continuous("Deadspace (ml)", limits=c(29,120),
      breaks=seq(30,120,10))+
    # Use the black and white theme with size 10 font
    theme_bw(base_size=10)+
    # Set the legend title, background and position
    theme(legend.title = element_blank(), legend.background = element_blank(),
    legend.position = c(0.15,0.9))+
    # Remove the major and minor grid lines
    theme(panel.grid.major = element_blank(), panel.grid.minor = element_blank())
```

Figure 2.2 Parallel slopes for children with and without asthma.

```
ggplot(data=Lung.Function,
    aes(x = Height, y = Deadspace, color = Asthma.Labels, shape =
      Asthma.Labels))+
    # Add the data points to the plot and set the colour for each group
    geom_point(size=2)+
    scale_colour_manual(values = c("Children without asthma"="black", "Children
      with asthma"="darkgrey"))+
    # Add the regression lines
    geom_smooth(method="lm",formula = y~x, se=F, fullrange=T, size=0.5)+
    # Label the x and y axes, setting the limits and breaks
    scale_x_continuous("Height (cm)", limits=c(110,180),
      breaks=seq(110,180,10))+
    scale_y_continuous("Deadspace (ml)", limits=c(29,120),
      breaks=seq(30,120,10))+
    # Use the black and white theme with size 10 font
    theme_bw(base_size=10)+
    # Set the legend title, background and position
    theme(legend.title = element_blank(), legend.background = element_blank(),
    legend.position = c(0.15,0.9))+
    # Remove the major and minor grid lines
    theme(panel.grid.major = element_blank(), panel.grid.minor = element_blank())
```

Figure 2.3 Separate lines for children with and without asthma.

Table 2.3 Output from computer program fitting height to deadspace for data from Table 2.1.

```
# Fit a linear regression model with Deadspace as the dependent variable and
# Height as the independent variable

    Model.2.1 <- lm(Deadspace ~ Height, data = Lung.Function)

# Print a summary of the model

    summary(Model.2.1)

# Calculate confidence intervals

    confint(Model.2.1)
```

Table 2.4 Results of fitting model 2.3 to the asthma data.

```
# Fit a linear regression model with Deadspace as the dependent variable
# and Height and Asthma as independent variables

    Model.2.2 <- lm(Deadspace ~ Height + Asthma, data = Lung.Function)

# Print a summary of the model

    summary(Model.2.2)

# Calculate confidence intervals

    confint(Model.2.2)
```

Table 2.5 Results of fitting model 2.4 to the asthma data.

```
# Fit a linear regression model with Deadspace as the dependent variable
# and Height, Asthma and the interaction between Height and Asthma as
# independent variables

    Model.2.3 <- lm(Deadspace ~ Height * Asthma, data = Lung.Function)

# Print a summary of the model

    summary(Model.2.3)

# Calculate confidence intervals

    confint(Model.2.3)
```

Table 2.6 Results of fitting model 2.5 to the asthma data.

```
# Fit a linear regression model with Deadspace as the dependent variable
# and Height and Age as the independent variables

    Model.2.4 <- lm(Deadspace ~ Height + Age, data = Lung.Function)

# Print a summary of the model

    summary(Model.2.4)

# Calculate confidence intervals

    confint(Model.2.4)
```

Table 2.7 Results using age and height standardised to have mean zero and standard deviation one.

```
# Calculate new variables for Deadspace, Height and Age with mean zero and
# standard deviation one

    Lung.Function$Deadspacestd <- scale(Lung.Function$Deadspace)
    Lung.Function$Heightstd <- scale(Lung.Function$Height)
    Lung.Function$Agestd <- scale(Lung.Function$Age)

# Fit a linear regression model with standardised Deadspace as the dependent
# variable and standardised Height and standardised Age as the independent
# variables

    Model.2.5 <- lm(Deadspacestd ~ Heightstd + Agestd, data = Lung.Function)

# Print a summary of the model

    summary(Model.2.5)

# Calculate confidence intervals

    confint(Model.2.5)
```

Table 2.8 Results of fitting asthma and bronchitis to deadspace.

```
# Fit a linear regression model with Deadspace as the dependent variable
# and Asthma and Bronchitis as the independent variables

    Model.2.6 <- lm(Deadspace ~ Asthma + Bronchitis, data = Lung.Function)

# Print a summary of the model

    summary(Model.2.6)

# Calculate confidence intervals

    confint(Model.2.6)

# An alternative method of fitting this model is to have a single factor
# variable (Status) with 0 = Normal, 1 = Asthma and 2 = Bronchitis

    Lung.Function$Status <- as.numeric(0)
    Lung.Function$Status[Lung.Function$Asthma == 1] <- 1
    Lung.Function$Status[Lung.Function$Bronchitis == 1] <- 2

    Lung.Function$Status <- factor(Lung.Function$Status,
                          levels = c(0,1,2),
                          labels = c("Normal", "Asthma", "Bronchitis"))

    Model.2.7 <- lm(Deadspace ~ Status, data = Lung.Function)
    summary(Model.2.7)

confint(Model.2.7)
```

Table 2.9 Results of fitting asthma and normal to deadspace.

```
# Create a variable indicating "Normal" status.

    Lung.Function$Normal <- c(0,0,0,0,0,1,0,0,0,0,0,0,0,1,1)

    Model.2.8 <- lm(Deadspace ~ Asthma + Normal, data = Lung.Function)

# Print a summary of the model

    summary(Model.2.8)

# Calculate confidence intervals

    confint(Model.2.8)

# An alternative method of fitting this model is to have a single factor
# variable as above but with Bronchitis as the first level of the factor

    Lung.Function$Status2 <- factor(Lung.Function$Status,
                               levels = c("Bronchitis", "Asthma", "Normal"))

    Model.2.9 <- lm(Deadspace ~ Status2, data = Lung.Function)

# Print a summary of the model

    summary(Model.2.9)

# Calculate confidence intervals

    confint(Model.2.9)
```

```
# Fit a linear regression model with Deadspace as the dependent
# variable and Height and Age as the independent variables

    Model.2.4 <- lm(Deadspace ~ Height + Age, data = Lung.Function)

# Create a data frame of the fitted values and residuals from the model

    Model.2.4.resid <- data.frame(Fitted.Values = fitted(Model.2.4),
                    Residuals = resid(Model.2.4))

# Plot the residuals on the y-axis against the fitted values on the x-axis

   ggplot(Model.2.4.resid, aes(x = Fitted.Values, y = Residuals))+
    geom_point()+
    scale_x_continuous("Fitted values", limits=c(0,120), breaks=seq(0,120,20))+
    scale_y_continuous("Residuals", limits=c(-25,25), breaks=seq(-20,20,10))+
    theme_bw(base_size=10)+
    theme(panel.grid.major = element_blank(), panel.grid.minor = element_blank())
```

Figure 2.4 Graph of residuals against fitted values for model 2.6 using age and height as independent variables.

Table 2.11 Diagnostics from model fitted to Table 2.4.

```
# Fit a linear regression model with Deadspace as the dependent variable
# and Height and Age as the independent variables

    Model.2.4 <- lm(Deadspace ~ Height + Age, data = Lung.Function)

# Calculate residuals

    Model.2.4.resid <- residuals(Model.2.4)

# Calculate leverage values

    Model.2.4.leverage <- hatvalues(Model.2.4)

# Calculate influence statistics

    Model.2.4.influence <- dfbetas(Model.2.4)

# Combine results into a data frame

    Model.2.4.diagnostics <- data.frame(Height = Lung.Function$Height,
                          Age = Lung.Function$Age,
                          resids = round(Model.2.4.resid, 2),
                          leverage = round(Model.2.4.leverage, 2),
                          inf_age = round(Model.2.4.influence[,3], 2),
                          inf_height = round(Model.2.4.influence[,2], 2))
```

A5.3 R Code for Chapter 3

R Libraries

The Hosmer-Lemeshow statistic is calculated using the ResourceSelection[3] library and the Epi[4] library is used conditional logistic regression

```
library(ResourceSelection)
library(Epi)
```

Table 3.2 Results for the Isoniazid trial after six months of follow-up.

Data for a grouped analysis

```
Isoniazid.Grouped.Data <-
    data.frame(Dead = c(21,11),
       Total = c (131, 132),
       Treatment = factor(c(0,1)))
```

Data for an ungrouped analysis

```
Isoniazid.Ungrouped.Data <-
    data.frame(Outcome = factor(rep(c(1,0,1,0), times = c(21,110,11,121))),
       Treatment = factor(rep(c(0,0,1,1), times = c(21,110,11,121))))
```

Table 3.3 Output from R logistic regression programs for grouped data from Table 3.2.

When using grouped data in R the outcome is two columns of data. The first representing the number of responses (in this case death) and the second representing the number of non-responses (in this case alive).

```
# Fit the null model. This model just contains a constant term.

    Model.3.1a <- glm(cbind(Dead,Total-Dead) ~ 1, family = binomial,
             data = Isoniazid.Grouped.Data)

# Print a summary of the model.

    summary(Model.3.1a)

# Fit the model with treatment group.

    Model.3.1b <- glm(cbind(Dead,Total-Dead) ~ Treatment, family = binomial,
             data = Isoniazid.Grouped.Data)

# Print a summary of the model.

    summary(Model.3.1b)

# Calculate odds ratio and 95% confidence interval for treatment.

exp(cbind(OR = Model.3.1b$coefficients, confint.default(Model.3.1b)))[-1,]
```

Table 3.4 Output from R logistic regression programs for ungrouped data from Table 3.2.

When using ungrouped data in R the outcome is a single variable indicating responses and non-responses.

```
# Fit the null model. This model just contains a constant term.
    Model.3.2a <- glm(Outcome ~ 1, family = binomial,
              data = Isoniazid.Ungrouped.Data)
# Print a summary of the model.
    summary(Model.3.2a)
# Fit the model with treatment group.
    Model.3.2b <- glm(Outcome ~ Treatment, family = binomial,
              data = Isoniazid.Ungrouped.Data)
# Print a summary of the model.
    summary(Model.3.2b)
# Calculate odds ratio and 95% confidence interval for treatment.
    exp(cbind(OR = Model.3.2b$coefficients, confint.default(Model.3.2b)))[-1,]
```

Table 3.6 Data from Julious and Mullee on mortality of diabetics.

```
Diabetes.Data <-
    data.frame(Dead = c(0,1,218,104),
      Total = c(15,130,529,228),
      Insulin_Dependent = c(0,1,0,1),
      Age = c(0,0,1,1))
```

Data from Julious SA, Mullee MA. Confounding and Simpson's Paradox. *Br Med J* 1994; **309**: 1480–1.

Table 3.7 Selected output for R program fitting logistic regression to Table 3.6.

```
# Fit model with Insulin_Dependent as a covariate
    Model.3.5 <- glm(cbind(Dead,Total-Dead) ~ Insulin_Dependent,
              family = binomial, data = Diabetes.Data)
# Print summary of the model
    summary(Model.3.5)
# Calculate odds ratios and 95% confidence intervals
      cbind(OR = exp(Model.3.5$coefficients),
        exp(confint.default(Model.3.5)),
        "Pr(>|z|)" = summary(Model.3.5)$coefficients[,4])[-1,]
# Fit model with Insulin_Dependent and Age as covariates
    Model.3.6 <- glm(cbind(Dead,Total-Dead) ~ Insulin_Dependent + Age,
              family = binomial, data = Diabetes.Data)
# Print summary of the model
    summary(Model.3.6)
# Calculate odds ratios and 95% confidence intervals
    cbind(OR = exp(Model.3.6$coefficients),
      exp(confint.default(Model.3.6)),
      "Pr(>|z|)" = summary(Model.3.6)$coefficients[,4])[-1,]
```

Table 3.8 Selection of R code to fit logistic regression to abdominal data.

Please note that the complications data is not available for download and this section of code is for illustration only.

```
# Read in the complications following abdominal operations data file

   Complications.Data <- read.csv("Complications.csv", header = T)

# Remove missing data for complete case analysis

   Complications.Data <- na.omit(Complications.Data)

# Fit logistic regression model with severity as the dependent variable and
# apache score and weight as the independent variables

   Model.3.7 <- glm(severity ~ apache + weight, family = binomial,
             data = Complications.Data)

# Print summary of the model

   summary(Model.3.7)

# Calculate odds ratios and 95% confidence intervals

     exp(cbind(OR = Model.3.7$coefficients, confint.default(Model.3.7)))[-1,]

# Calculate LR chi2

     with(Model.3.7, null.deviance - deviance)

# Calculate Prob > chi2

     with(Model.3.7, pchisq(null.deviance - deviance, df.null - df.residual,
               lower.tail = FALSE))

# Calculate Hosmer-Lemeshow

     hoslem.test(Model.3.7$y, fitted(Model.3.7))
```

Table 3.10 Exposure to passive smoking among female lung cancer cases and controls in four studies.

```
Case.Control.Unmatched <-
   data.frame(Cases = c(14,8,33,8,13,11,91,43),
     N = c(75,80,197,40,28,21,345,191),
     Exposed = factor(c(1,0,1,0,1,0,1,0)),
     Study = factor(c(1,1,2,2,3,3,4,4)))
```

Data from Wald NJ, Nanchahal K, Thompson SG, Cuckle HS. Does breathing other people's tobacco smoke cause lung cancer? *Br Med J* 1986; **293**: 1217–22.

Table 3.11 Output from a logistic regression program for the case-control study in Table 3.10.

```
# Fit logistic regression model on grouped data with study and exposed as
# independent variables

   Model.3.8 <- glm(cbind(Cases,N-Cases) ~ Study + Exposed, family = binomial,

            data = Case.Control.Unmatched)

# Print summary of the model

   summary(Model.3.8)

# Calculate odds ratios and 95% confidence intervals

   exp(cbind(OR = Model.3.8$coefficients, confint.default(Model.3.8)))[-1,]
```

Table 3.12 Adequacy of monitoring in hospital of 35 deaths and 35 matched survivors with asthma.

```
Case.Control.Matched <-
    data.frame(Pair = rep(c(1:35), each = 2),
       Case.Control = rep(c(1,0), 35),
       Monitoring = c(rep(1,20), rep(c(1,0), 13), rep(c(0,1), 3), rep(0,18)))
```

Adapted from Eason J, Markowe HLJ. Controlled investigation of deaths from asthma in hospitals in the North East Thames region. *Br Med J* 1987; **294**: 1255–8.

Table 3.14 Output from conditional logistic regression of the matched case-control study in Table 3.12.

```
# Fit conditional logistic regression model.
# Case.Control (1=death, 0=survival) is the dependent variable
# Monitoring is the independent variable and pair is the strata

    Model.3.9 <- clogistic(Case.Control ~ Monitoring, strata = Pair,
             data = Case.Control.Matched)

# Print summary of the model

    Model.3.9

# Calculate odds ratios and 95% confidence intervals

    exp(cbind(OR = Model.3.9$coefficients, confint(Model.3.9)))
```

A5.4 R Code for Chapter 4

R Libraries

The Kaplan-Meier curves and Cox proportional hazard models are fit using the survival library,[5,6] Kaplan-Meier plots and complementary log-log plots are drawn using the survminer[7] library.

```
library(survival)
library(survminer)
```

Table 4.1 Survival in 49 patients with Dukes' C colorectal cancer randomly assigned to either linolenic acid or control treatment.

```
Survival.Data <-
 data.frame(
Time=c(1,5,6,6,9,10,10,10,12,12,12,12,12,13,15,16,20,24,24,27,32,34,36,36,44,3,6,
   6,6,6,8,8,12,12,12,15,16,18,18,20,22,24,28,28,28,30,30,33,42),
Event=c(0,0,1,1,0,1,1,0,1,1,1,1,0,0,0,0,0,1,0,0,1,0,0,0,0,0,1,1,1,1,1,1,1,1,0,0,
   0,0,0,1,0,1,0,0,0,1,0,0,1),
Group=factor(rep(c(1,0), times = c(25,24))))
```

```
# Create a variable for the names of the treatment groups
    Survival.Data$Group.Name <- factor(Survival.Data$Group)
    levels(Survival.Data$Group.Name)[1] <- "Control"
    levels(Survival.Data$Group.Name)[2] <- "Linolenic Acid"
# Fit a Kaplan-Meier curve for each treatment group
    KM.curves <- survfit(Surv(Time,Event) ~ Group.Name, data = Survival.Data)
# Change the attributes of the curves so that the group names match the
# levels of the variable
    attr(KM.curves$strata,"names") <- levels(Survival.Data$Group.Name)
# Plot the Kaplan-Meier curves with number at risk table
    ggsurvplot(KM.curves, data = Survival.Data, risk.table = TRUE,
    palette=c("gray60", "black"), legend.title = "Group")
```

Figure 4.1 Kaplan-Meier survival plots for data in Table 4.1.

Table 4.2 Analysis of linolenic acid data.

```
# Fit a Cox proportional hazard model using the exact partial likelihood
# method for handling ties
   Model.4.1 <- coxph(Surv(Time,Event) ~ Group, data = Survival.Data,
      ties="exact")
# Print a summary of the model
   summary(Model.4.1)
# Calculate the log likelihood
   logLik(Model.4.1)
```

```
# Fit a Kaplan-Meier curve for each treatment group
    KM.curves <- survfit(Surv(Time,Event) ~ Group.Name, data = Survival.Data)
# Change the attributes of the curves so that the group names match the
# levels of the variable
    attr(KM.curves$strata,"names") <- levels(Survival.Data$Group.Name)
# Plot the complementary log-log plot
    ggsurvplot(KM.curves, data = Survival.Data,
       fun = "cloglog",
       censor = FALSE,
       xlab = "Time (Months)",
       ylab = "ln(-ln(Survival Probability)",
       palette=c("gray60", "black"),
       ggtheme = theme_bw(),
       legend.title = "Group",
       legend = c(0.15,0.9))
```

Figure 4.2 Log-log plot of survival curves in Figure 4.1.

Table 4.3 Test of proportional hazards assumption

```
cox.zph(Model.4.1, global = TRUE)
```

A5.5 R Code for Chapter 5

R Libraries

Linear regression models with cluster robust standard errors are fit using the estimatr[8] library. Maximum likelihood random effects models are fit using the lme4[9] library with p-values and confidence intervals calculated using the lmerTest[10] library. Linear models using generalised estimating equations are fit using the geepack[11] library. The tidyverse[12] library is used to summarise the BMI data before fitting a model using group means.

```
library(estimatr)
library(lme4)
library(lmerTest)
library(geepack)
library(tidyverse)
```

Table 5.1 Data on BMI.

```
BMI.Data <-
    data.frame(ID = c(1:20),
       BMI = c(26.2,27.1,25.0,28.3,30.5,28.8,31.0,32.1,28.2,30.9,37.0,38.1,22.1,
          23.0,23.2,25.7,27.8,28.0,28.0,31.0),
       Treatment = rep(c(1,0), each = 10),
       Practice = factor(c(1,1,2,2,3,4,4,4,5,5,6,6,7,7,8,8,9,9,10,10)))
```

Data from Kinmonth AL, Woodcock A, Griffin S, Spiegal N, Campbell MJ. Randomised controlled trial of patient centred care of diabetes in general practice: impact on current well-being and future disease risk. *BMJ* 1988; **317**: 1202-08.

Table 5.2 (i) Regression not allowing for clustering.

```
# Fit linear regression model
    Model.5.2.1 <- lm(BMI ~ Treatment, data = BMI.Data)
# Print a summary of the model
    summary(Model.5.2.1)
# Calculate confidence intervals
    confint(Model.5.2.1)
```

Table 5.2 (ii) Regression with robust SEs.

```
# Fit regression model specifying Practice as clusters and robust standard
# error type as "CR2"
    Model.5.2.2 <- lm_robust(BMI ~ Treatment, data = BMI.Data,
    clusters = Practice, se_type = "CR2")
# Print a summary of the model
    summary(Model.5.2.2)
```

Table 5.2 (iii) Maximum likelihood random effects model.

```
# Fit maximum likelihood random effects model with Practice as the random
# intercept

   Model.5.2.3 <- lmer(BMI ~ Treatment + (1 | Practice), data = BMI.Data,
      REML=F)

# Print a summary of the model

   summary(Model.5.2.3)

# Calculate profile based confidence intervals for the fixed effects

   confint(Model.5.2.3, parm = c("(Intercept)","Treatment"))
```

Table 5.2 (iv) Generalised estimating equations.

```
# Fit linear regression model using generalised estimating equations
# specifying Practice as the cluster id and an exchangeable correlation
# structure

   Model.5.2.4 <- geeglm(BMI ~ Treatment, id=Practice, corstr="exchangeable",

   data = BMI.Data)

# Print a summary of the model

   summary(Model.5.2.4)

# Calculate confidence intervals

   lower <-

   coef(summary(Model.5.2.4))[,1]+qnorm(0.025)*coef(summary(Model.5.2.4))[,2]

   upper <-

   coef(summary(Model.5.2.4))[,1]+qnorm(0.975)*coef(summary(Model.5.2.4))[,2]

   cbind(coef(summary(Model.5.2.4)), lower, upper)
```

Table 5.2 (v) Regression on group means.

```
# Summarise the BMI data calculating the mean for each Practice

   BMI.Summary <-
   BMI.Data %>%
   group_by(Practice, Treatment) %>%
   summarise(BMI.Mean = mean(BMI), .groups = "drop")

# Fit a linear regression model with mean BMI as the dependent variable

   Model.5.2.5 <- lm(BMI.Mean ~ Treatment, data = BMI.Summary)

# Print a summary of the model

   summary(Model.5.2.5)

# Calculate confidence intervals

   confint(Model.5.2.5)
```

A5.6 R Code for Chapter 6

R Libraries

Robust standard errors are calculated using the sandwich[13,14] library and applied using the lmtest[15] library. The ordinal[16] library is used for ordinal regression.

```
library(sandwich)
library(lmtest)
library(ordinal)
```

Table 6.1 Coronary deaths from British male doctors.

```
Deaths <- c(32,2,104,12,206,28,186,28,102,31)
    Person.Years <- c(52407,18790,43248,10673,28612,5712,12663,2585,5317,1462)
    Smoker <- factor(rep(c(1,0),5))
    Age.Group <-
      factor(rep(c("35-44","45-54","55-64","65-74","75-84"),each=2))
    Coronary.Deaths <- data.frame(Deaths,Person.Years,Smoker,Age.Group)
```

Table 6.2 Results of Poisson regression on data in Table 6.1.

```
# Fit a Poisson regression model with Deaths as the dependent variable and
# Smoker and Age.Group as independent variables. The offset is the natural
# log of Person.Years
    Model.6.1 <- glm(Deaths ~ Smoker + Age.Group, offset = log(Person.Years),
             family = "poisson", data = Coronary.Deaths)
# Print a summary of the model
    summary(Model.6.1)
# Extract IRRs for Smoker and Age.Group by taking exponential of the
# coefficients and calculate confidence intervals
    exp(cbind(IRR = Model.6.1$coefficients, confint.default(Model.6.1)))[-1,]
```

Table 6.3 Using Poisson regression to estimate a relative risk, as a substitute for logistic regression.

```
# Create the ungrouped Isoniazid data
    Isoniazid.Ungrouped.Data <-
    data.frame(Outcome = rep(c(1,0,1,0), times = c(21,110,11,121)),
      Treatment = factor(rep(c(0,0,1,1), times = c(21,110,11,121))))
# Fit a Poisson regression model with Outcome as the dependent variable and
# Treatment as the independent variable
    Model.6.2 <- glm(Outcome ~ Treatment, family = "poisson",
             data = Isoniazid.Ungrouped.Data)
# Robust standard errors HC3
    Model.6.2.robust <- coeftest(Model.6.2,vcov=vcovHC(Model.6.2,type="HC3"))
# Print a summary of the model
    Model.6.2.robust
# Calculate IRR and 95% CI for Treatment
    IRR <- exp(coef(Model.6.2.robust))
    CI <- exp(coefci(Model.6.2,vcov=vcovHC(Model.6.2,type="HC3")))
```

Table 6.4 Change in eating poultry in randomised trial.

```
# Create the change in eating habits data

    Eating.Habits <-
      data.frame(Outcome = factor(rep(c(1,2,3,1,2,3),
      times = c(42,175,100,59,173,78))),

      Group = factor(rep(c(1,0), times = c(317,310))))
```

Data from Cupples ME, McKnight A. Randomised controlled trial of health promotions in general practice for patients at high cardiovascular risk. *BMJ* 1994; **309**: 993-96.

Table 6.5 Results of ordinal regression in Table 6.4.

```
# Fit ordinal logistic regression model with Outcome as the dependent
# variable and Group as the independent variable
    Model.6.3 <- clm2(Outcome ~ Group, data = Eating.Habits)
# Print a summary of the model
    summary(Model.6.3)
# Calculate odds ratio and 95% CI
    exp(cbind(OR = Model.6.3$coefficients, confint.default(Model.6.3)))[3,]
```

A5.7 R Code for Chapter 7

R Libraries

Meta-analysis is conducted using the meta[17] library.

```
library(meta)
```

Data from Gera and Sachdev

```
# Create vector showing study names
study<-c("James", "Brusner", "Fuerth", "Menendez 1", "Menendez 2", "Hombergh",
   "Angeles", "Power", "Palupi", "Rosado 1", "Rosado 2", "Javaid", "Berger",
   "Lawless", "Irigoyen", "Oppenheimer", "Singhal", "Mitra", "Hemminki", "Agar-
   wal", "Nagpal", "Rice", "Idjradinata", "Smith", "Adam", "Gabresellasie",
   "Atukorala 1", "Atukorala 2", "Cantwell")
# Create vectors of outcomes
# a = number of events for exposed
a <- c(96,256,1007,75,36,107,9,469,71,285,202,432,1328,26,20,1027,889,1375,504,
   12,3,2781,19,14,176,219,297,137,15)
# b = exposure time for exposed
b <- c(77,56.88,493.5,118.4,148.5,12.5,6.5,52.5,15.5,54,55,58,75,11,114,196.66,
   121.5,134,164,3.75,4.5,267.97,8,26.5,107.75,187.5,21.33,22.33,188)
# c = number of events for control
c <- c(116,254,773,81,42,65,21,460,69,255,211,189,1178,26,13,921,2001,1420,521,
   5,3,2798,21,8,146,206,147,70,44)
# d = exposure time for controls
d <- c(88.91,72.57,409.5,113.8,145.4,12.5,6.16,46.5,15.66,56,54,28,72.75,10.5,53
   ,208.33,248.25,143.5,158,3.58,5,267.39,7.66,26.75,102.5,187.5,8.66,8.33,288)
```

Table 7.1 Analysis of data from Gera and Sachdev.

```
# Fixed and random effects meta-analysis
    model.7.1 <-
    metainc(event.e = a, time.e = b, event.c = c, time.c = d, studlab = study,
    sm = "IRR", method = "inverse", method.tau = "REML", prediction = T)
# Print results
    model.7.1
```

```
# Forest plot using results from model 7.1

    forest.meta(model.7.1, fixed = F, pooled.events = T, pooled.times = T,
    label.e = "Iron", label.c = "Control",
    digits.time = 0, print.I2 = F, print.Q = T, print.tau2 = F,
    digits.pval.Q = 4, xlim = c(0.1,10),
    col.diamond.random = "black", col.inside = "black")
```

Figure 7.1 A forest plot for the incidence rate ratio for infection in trials of iron supplementation in children for all infectious diseases.
Gera T, Sachdev HP. Effect of iron supplementation on incidence of infectious illness in children: a systematic review. *BMJ* 2002; **325**: 1142–51. https://www.bmj.com/content/325/7373/1142

Table 7.2 Using Poisson regression to carry out a fixed effect analysis of data from Figure 7.1.

```
# Format data for Poisson model

# Outcome data
    y <- c(a,c)
# Exposure time data
    e <- c(b,d)
# Exposure/control variable
    iron <- rep(c(1,0),c(length(a),length(c)))
# Study variable
    studyf <- factor(rep(study,2))

# fit Poisson model
    model.7.2 <- glm(y ~ iron + studyf, family = poisson, offset = log(e))

# Print summary of the model

    summary(model.7.2)

# Calculate IRR and confidence interval for exposure

    exp(cbind(IRR = model.7.2$coefficients, confint.default(model.7.2)))[2,]
```

```
funnel(model.7.1, yaxis = "invse", backtransf = FALSE)
```

Figure 7.2 A funnel plot for the iron supplementation study of Gera and Sachdev.
Gera T, Sachdev HP. Effect of iron supplementation on incidence of infectious illness in children: a systematic review. *BMJ* 2002; **325**: 1142–51.https://www.bmj.com/content/325/7373/1142

A5.8 R Code for Chapter 8

R Libraries

Time series regression models using the Cochrane-Orcutt procedure are fit using the orcutt[18] library.

```
library(orcutt)
```

Table 8.1 Results of Cochrane-Orcutt regression of deadspace against height on the data in Table 2.1 assuming points all belong to one individual over time.

```
# Create a data frame of the lung function data

    Lung.Function <-
      data.frame(Child.Number = c(1:15),
         Deadspace = c(44,31,43,45,56,79,57,56,58,92,78,64,88,112,101),
         Height = c(110,116,124,129,131,138,142,150,153,155,156,159,164,168,174),
         Asthma = c(1,0,1,1,1,0,1,1,1,0,0,1,0,0,0),
         Age = c(5,5,6,7,7,6,6,8,8,9,7,8,10,11,14),
         Bronchitis = c(0,1,0,0,0,0,0,0,0,1,1,0,1,0,0))

# Analysis not allowing for autocorrelation
# Fit a linear regression model with Deadspace as the dependent variable and
# Height as the independent variable

    Model.8.1 <- lm(Deadspace ~ Height, data = Lung.Function)

# Print a summary of the model

    summary(Model.8.1)

# Analysis allowing for autocorrelation

    Model.8.2 <- cochrane.orcutt(Model.8.1)

# Print a summary of the model

    summary(Model.8.2)
```

A5.9 R Code for Appendix 1

R Libraries

Plots are drawn using the ggplot[1] library.

```
library(ggplot2)
```

```
# Create function to be used in plot
    log_fn <- function(x){log(x)}
# Plot the function
    ggplot(data.frame(x = c(0.1, 10)), aes(x=x))+
    # Add the log_fn function to the plot
    stat_function(fun=log_fn)+
    # label the y-axis
    scale_y_continuous("log to base e of x")+
    # label the x-axis and set breaks
    scale_x_continuous("x", breaks = seq(0,10,2))+
    # Use the black and white theme with size 12 font
    theme_bw(base_size=12)+
    # Remove the major and minor grid lines
    theme(panel.grid.major = element_blank(), panel.grid.minor = element_
       blank())
```

Figure A1.1 $\text{Log}_e(x)$ vs x.

A5.10 R Code for Appendix 2

R Libraries

Plots are drawn using the ggplot[1] library.

```
library(ggplot2)
```

```
# Create function to be used in plot
    binomial <- function(x){2*log(x) + 3*log(1-x) }

# Plot the function

    ggplot(data.frame(x = c(0.001, 0.999)), aes(x=x))+
    # Add the binomial function to the plot
    stat_function(fun=binomial)+
    # Label the y-axis
    scale_y_continuous("Log-likelihood", limits=c(-15,0))+
    # Label the x-axis
    scale_x_continuous(expression(pi), breaks = seq(0,1,0.1))+
    # Use black and white theme with size 12 font
    theme_bw(base_size=12)+
    # Remove the major and minor grid lines
    theme(panel.grid.major = element_blank(), panel.grid.minor = element_blank())
```

Figure A2.1 Graph of log-likelihood against π, for a Binomial model with D=2 and N=5.

```
# Create function to be used in plot
    normal <- function(x){ (-10/2)*(((175-x)^2)/15)}
# Plot the function

    ggplot(data.frame(x = c(145, 205)), aes(x=x))+
      # Add the binomial function to the plot
      stat_function(fun=normal)+
      # Label the y-axis
      scale_y_continuous("Log-likelihood", breaks = seq(-300,0,50))+
      # Label the x-axis
      scale_x_continuous(expression(mu), breaks = seq(145,205,5))+
      # Use black and white theme with size 12 font
      theme_bw(base_size=12)+
      # Remove the major and minor grid lines
      theme(panel.grid.major = element_blank(), panel.grid.minor = element_blank())
```

Figure A2.2 Graph of log-likelihood of a single observation from a Normal model.

A5.11 R Code for Appendix 3

R Libraries

The simpleboot[19] library is used for bootstrapping the median of a single sample and the car[20] library is used for bootstrapping the residuals of a linear regression model. Bootstrap confidence intervals are calculated using the boot[21,22] library. The broom[23] library is used for formatting the output of the independent samples t-test. Robust standard errors are calculated using the sandwich[13,14] library and applied using the lmtest[15] library.

```
library(simpleboot)
library(boot)
library(car)
library(broom)
library(lmtest)
library(sandwich)
```

Table A3.1 Calculating a bootstrap confidence interval for a median.

```
# Create a vector for the original beta-endorphin concentrations sample

    beta.endorphin <- c(66, 71.2, 83.0, 83.6, 101, 107.6, 122, 143, 160,  177, 414)

# Set seed to give identical output

    set.seed(100)

# Bootstrap the median with 1000 replicates

    median.boot <- one.boot(beta.endorphin, median, R=1000)

# Calculate confidence intervals

    boot.ci(median.boot, type = c("norm","perc","bca"))
```

Table A3.2 Output illustrating use of the bootstrap to compare two means.

```
# Deadspace data

    a1 <- c(43,44,45,56,56,57,58,64)
    a2 <- c(31,78,79,88,92,101,112)
    Deadspace <- c(a1,a2)
    Asthma <- c(rep(1,length(a1)),rep(0,length(a2)))
    Lung.Function <- data.frame(Deadspace,Asthma)
```

(i) Two-sample t-test with equal variances

```
# Two sample t-test with equal variances

    t_equal_res <- t.test(a1, a2, var.equal = T)

# Calculate difference in means

    diff<-mean(a1)-mean(a2)

# Print the results

    t_equal_res

cat("Difference in means", diff)

cat("Standard deviations with and without asthma", sd(a1),sd(a2))
```

(ii) Bootstrap confidence interval

```
# Fit a linear model with Deadspace as the dependent variable and Asthma
# as the independent variable
    fit <- lm(Deadspace ~ Asthma, data = Lung.Function)
# Bootstap the residuals
# The function f extracts the coefficient estimate for treatment
# The bootstrapping is stratified by Asthma status
# Set seed to give identical output
    set.seed(100)
    lm.boot <- Boot(fit, f=function(obj){coef(obj)[2]}, R=1000,
    method="residual", strata=Asthma)
# Print a summary of the bootstrap
    summary(lm.boot)
# Calculate bootstrap confidence intervals
    boot.ci(lm.boot, type = c("norm","perc","bca"))
```

Table A3.3 Computer output using robust regression for unequal variances.

(i) Two-sample t-test with unequal variances

```
t_unequal_res <- t.test(a1, a2, var.equal = F)
# Print results
    t_unequal_res
```

(ii) Regression with robust standard errors: HC0

```
# Calculate degrees of freedom
    n1<-length(a1)
    n2<-length(a2)
    v1<-var(a1)
    v2<-var(a2)
    df<-(v1/n1+v2/n2)^2/(((v1/n1)^2)/(n1-1)+(((v2/n2)^2)/(n2-1)))
# Fit model
    mod_glm <- glm(Deadspace ~ Asthma, data = Lung.Function,
                   family=gaussian(link="identity"))
# Robust standard error HC0
    mhc0<-coeftest(mod_glm, df=df, vcov = vcovHC(mod_glm, type="HC0"))
# Print a summary of the model
    mhc0
# Calculate confidence intervals
    confint(mhc0)
```

(iii) Regression with robust standard errors: HC2

```
mhc2<-coeftest(mod_glm, df=df, vcov = vcovHC(mod_glm, type="HC2"))
# Print a summary of the model
    mhc2
# Calculate confidence intervals
    confint(mhc2)
```

(iv) Regression with robust standard errors: HC3

```
mch3<-coeftest(mod_glm, df=df, vcov = vcovHC(mod_glm, type="HC3"))
# Print a summary of the model
    mch3
# Calculate confidence intervals
    confint(mhc3)
```

References

1 Wickham H. ggplot2: *elegant Graphics for Data Analysis*. New York: Springer-Verlag, 2016.

2 Kim AY, Ismay C, Kuhn M. Take a moderndive into introductory linear regression with R. *Journal of Open Source Education* 2021; **4**(21): 115. https://doi.org/10.21105/jose.00115.

3 Lele SR, Keim JL, Solymos P. Resource selection (probability) functions for use-availability data. R package version 0.3-5. https://CRAN.R-project.org/package=ResourceSelection

4 Carstensen B, Plummer M, Laara E, Hills M. Epi: a package for statistical analysis in epidemiology. R package version 2.46. https://CRAN.R-project.org/package=Epi.

5 Therneau T. A package for survival analysis in R. R package version 3.2-11. https://CRAN.R-project.org/package=survival

6 Therneau TM, Grambsch PM. *Modeling Survival Data: Extending the Cox Model*. New York: Springer-Verlag, 2000.

7 Kassambara A, Kosinski M, Biecek P. survminer: drawing survival curves using 'ggplot2'. R package version 0.4.9. https://CRAN.R-project.org/package=survminer

8 Blair G, Cooper J, Coppock A, *et al*. estimatr: fast estimators for design-based inference. R package version 0.30.2. https://CRAN.R-project.org/package=estimatr

9 Bates D, Maechler M, Bolker B, *et al*. Fitting linear mixed-effects models using lme4. *Journal of Statistical Software* 2015; **67**(1): 1–48.

10 Kuznetsova A, Brockhoff PB, Christensen RHB. lmerTest package: tests in linear mixed effects models. *Journal of Statistical Software* 2017; **82**(13): 1–26.

11 Højsgaard S, Halekoh U, Yan J. The R package for generalized estimating equations. *Journal of Statistical Software* 2006; **15**(2): 1–11.

12 Wickham H, Averick M, Bryan J, *et al*. Welcome to the tidyverse. *Journal of Open Source Software* 2019; **4**(43): 1686.

13 Zeileis A. Object-oriented computation of sandwich estimators. *Journal of Statistical Software* 2006; **16**(9): 1–16. https://doi.org/10.18637/jss.v016.i09.

14 Zeileis A, Köll S, Graham N. Various versatile variances: an object-oriented implementation of clustered covariances in R. *Journal of Statistical Software* 2020; **95**(1): 1–36. https://doi.org/10.18637/jss.v095.i011.

15 Zeileis A, Hothorn T. Diagnostic checking in regression relationships. R News 2022; **2**(3): 7–10. https://CRAN.R-project.org/doc/Rnews

16 Christensen RHB. ordinal-regression models for ordinal data. R package version 2019.12-10. https://CRAN.R-project.org/package=ordinal.

17 Balduzzi S, Rücker G, Schwarzer G. How to perform a meta-analysis with R: a practical tutorial. *Evidence-Based Mental Health* 2019; **22**: 153–60.

18 Stefano S, Quartagno M, Tamburini M, Robinson D. orcutt: estimate procedure in case of first order autocorrelation. https://CRAN.R-project.org/package=orcutt

19 Peng RD. simpleboot: simple bootstrap routines. R package version 1.1-7. https://CRAN.R-project.org/package=simpleboot

20 Fox J, Weisberg S. *An R Companion to Applied Regression*, 3rd edn. Thousand Oaks CA: Sage, 2018.

21 Davison AC, Hinkley DV. *Bootstrap Methods and Their Applications*. Cambridge: Cambridge University Press, 1997.

22 Canty A, Ripley B. boot: bootstrap R (S-PLUS) functions. R package version 1.3-28. https://CRAN.R-project.org/package=boot

23 Robinson D, Hayes A, Couch S. broom: convert statistical objects into tidy tibbles. R package version 0.7.9. https://CRAN.R-project.org/package=broom

Answers to Exercises

Chapter 2

Exercise 2.1

a) The assumptions are.
   i) there is a linear relation between baseline and outcome;
   ii) acupuncture reduces the number of days of headache irrespective of the baseline value (i.e. treatment effect is the same for all subjects);
   iii) the residuals from the model are independent and approximately Normally distributed with constant variance.
b) The SD for these data is large relative to the mean, which suggests that in fact the data are likely to be skewed. The data are also restricted to a minimum of 0 and a maximum of 28, which also might lead to skewness. However, the mean values are close to centre of the range and sample size is quite large so the *p*-value is unlikely to be materially changed.
c) The CI for the analysis of covariance is larger than for the F-test. This suggests that there is only a loose association between the baseline and follow-up and so introducing a covariate has actually increased the SE. Note that the numbers of patients at baseline is not the same as that at follow-up, so we do not know if those who were followed up were comparable at baseline.
d) One might like to see: a plot of the distribution of the data, a plot of baseline vs follow-up for the two groups as in Figure 2.2 and the baseline values for those actually followed up. One might also like to see if, at baseline, the drop-outs differed from those who were subsequently followed up. A dot plot of the residuals by treatment group would help confirm whether they are plausibly Normally distributed with similar variance in the two groups.
e) The inclusion of the baseline did not change the results much because the treatment and control group were comparable at baseline, although what matters is whether those who were followed up are comparable at baseline.

Statistics at Square Two: Understanding Modern Statistical Application in Medicine, Third Edition.
Michael J. Campbell and Richard M. Jacques.

Exercise 2.2

a) Having an epidural is less satisfactory than having no anaesthetic, or other types of anaesthesia. Having a peri-urethral tear leads to more satisfaction (not having given birth the authors are not in a position to comment, but it seems odd). Readers can discuss. For every unit of time in total labour (not specified by given as hours elsewhere in the paper) satisfaction drops by 0.01. The t-statistic should be the ratio of B to SE(B) and looks odd unless there has been heavy rounding. Having a third degree perineal tear leads to much worse satisfaction.
b) The overall p-value of 0.045, suggests that the model is only slightly better than chance of explaining the data.
c) The standardised coefficient suggest that the most important factor in the model is having an epidural.
d) The model assumes that satisfaction goes down linearly with labour length, although the authors do not verify this.
e) The problem with stepwise regression is, as explained in section 2.8, the meaning of the coefficient changes when other categories are dropped, so epidural is now contrasted with combined other anaesthesia and none.
f) The third degree tears are compared to all those without third degree tears which includes those with first and second as well as no tears.
g) The length of first stage and second stage labour are clearly highly correlated with the total length of labour. The model suggests that if you know the total length of labour, the length of the first and second stage don't give additional information about satisfaction.
h) The R^2 of 19.4% suggests that the model explains little of mothers' satisfaction.

Chapter 3

1) Crude OR = (2097 × (2830 − 2788))/(2788 × (2136 − 2097)) = 0.81. Very close to the adjusted value, suggesting there was little imbalance in the covariates by gender.
2) The crude Relative Risk = (2097 × 2830)/(2788 × 2136) = 1.0. This suggests there was little difference between males and females. (The weighted values given in the paper were 82.5/83.8 = 0.98.)
3) The 95% CI for the OR for females relative to males does not include 1, suggesting that females were statistically significantly less likely than males to accept vaccination. This should be moderated by the fact that it was one of many tests.
4) The overall chi-squared statistic is not significant. It has 2 d.f. because it includes a third category "Other". Including this category, with very few numbers has the effect of lowering the power of the test and means the chi-squared test is not reliable.

Chapter 4 Survival

Exercise 4.1

a) There are 9 + 2 + 6 + 5 + 9 + 10 = 41 categories and 9 x 2 x 6 x 5 x 9 x10 = 48,600 strata. They could only fit this number of strata because they had such a large sample size. Note that because stratified Cox regression is a conditional model (similar to conditional logistic regression) no parameters are estimated for any of the variables that form the strata – these are instead treated as nuisance parameters and conditioned on.

b) The crude relative risk for the overall model is 4.7/3.5 = 1.34 compared to 1.51 for the adjusted model. The difference is likely due to differences in the confounders between those with/without Alpha. The authors comment that most of the Alpha variant occurred in the South and East of England and later in the follow-up period.

c) For an informal assessment one could say there was a statistically significant difference for people aged 20–29 to those overall, because the CIs don't overlap. However, the comparison is not strictly valid because the two groups are not completely independent, but this is only strictly valid if it is the only comparison.

d) The authors state that they used Schoenfeld tests to test for deviation from the proportional hazard assumption, and they visually assessed the assumption by examining log-log transformed Kaplan–Meier plots for Alpha status and each potential confounder. The plots (which were given in the supplementary material) show only small departures from proportional hazards. In addition, the authors show that there are no significant interactions between Covid type and covariates other than age, so the results are plausible.

e) No, for example the results are given by each age category as well as overall and so do not require any assumption about the relationship between age and hazard, such as a linearly increasing risk. Also the authors have shown that for other hazards the hazards are approximately proportional.

f) The number of censored observations are not given, but it is assumed to be all those not admitted by 14 days and those who died.

g) No, just the absolute risks for each variant group. However, this is useful information, because it shows the absolute risk to be low, especially for those aged 20–29.

Exercise 4.2

a) A stratified analysis was used because the authors wished to allow for possible differences in the ages of the exposed and non-exposed groups, but did not wish to assume a particular model for age. A stratified analysis assumes the risk is the same for each person within a ten-year age cohort, and that this risk may vary as the cohort ages. However, a person within a different ten-year cohort may have a different risk profile as they age.

b) The fact that the hazard ratio changes little when smoking is included in the model suggests that the groups are well matched for smoking habit. The fact that the hazard is reduced when FEV1 is included suggests that perhaps the slate workers were already suffering with a low FEV1 at baseline, and so FEV1 and slate exposure are not independent covariates.
c) Two major assumptions in model 2 are the proportional hazards assumption, which means that the risk of slate exposure remains constant over the 24 years, and a lack of interaction assumption, which means the effect of slate is the same whether or not the man is a smoker. The former could be examined by the log-log survival plot as described in Chapter 4 and the latter by fitting interaction terms in the model.
d) The interpretation of the coefficient associated with FEV1 is that for two people who are in the same ten-year age group, exposure category and smoking category, one with an FEV1 1 greater than the other has a risk of death of 74% compared to the other.

Chapter 5

Exercise 5.1

a) Patients are the random effect since a different trial will have different patients.
b) Treatment is a fixed effect which we want to estimate.
c) Age group is a fixed effect which we control for.
d) Smoking group is a fixed effect which we want to control for
e) Height is a fixed effect which we control for.
f) Measurements within patients are part of the random error, that is, we expect differences within patients to be purely random.

Exercise 5.2

a) Counsellors are the random effect since a different trial would have different counsellors.
b) Type of therapy is a fixed effect that we want to estimate.
c) Level of depression is a fixed effect that we want to control for.
d) Patients are the random error.

Exercise 5.3

a) The problems are that the authors have dichotomised a continuous variable and we would like to be reassured that this was done prior to examining the data. Also, dichotomising a continuous variable can result in loss of information. It might lead to a more sensitive analysis if the time to progression was taken into account. Two advantages are: simplicity in summarising the data and that they could combine two outcomes, a continuous one (joint space narrowing) and a discrete one (hip replacement).

b) The assumptions are that age is linearly related to the log odds ratio for all ages.
c) There is no interaction between age and sex, and the error is an over-dispersed binomial. The increase in the OR for 1 year is 1.06 and so we simply raise this to the power 10 to get the OR as 1.6 in someone 10 years older. It is the same for the 65- vs 75-year-olds; this is a consequence of the model.
d) We have to solve the equation $(\pi/(1 - \pi)/((0.13/0.87)) = 1.8$. This leads to $\pi = 0.21$ or about 21% of women are expected to progress.

Chapter 6

Exercise 6.1

a) The potential confounders were categorised so that the investigators could count the number of events and the exposure time in each category. If any of the confounders were continuous, then the number of events would be 0 or 1.
b) In fact the model is a *log-linear* one so one would expect a plot of the *log* of the incidence rates to be linearly related to the birth weight. In practice it might be difficult to distinguish between a linear and a log plot.
c) One could examine whether the data were over-dispersed and if so, the SEs would need adjustment.
d) Since time from birth to a diagnosis of diabetes is like a survival time, one could employ Cox regression as described in Chapter 4.

Exercise 6.2

a) The main outcome is an ordinal variable since we can assume that "too early" is a response between "at the right age" and "should not have happened", but we cannot assign ranks to these categories.
b) The authors used ordinal regression. It would be better than logistic regression because it does not require a dichotomy in the outcome, and if the assumptions are met, will prove to be more powerful. A multivariate model is necessary to see if the outcome is affected by confounders such as social class and parenting style.
c) The main assumption is one of proportional odds between the categories and the authors state they checked this. Without allowing for covariates this could be checked informally as follows. For girls the percentages in the three groups are 55;32;13 and for boys they are 68;27;5. Pooling the second and third categories the percentages are 55;45 for girls and 68;30, and pooling the first and second they are 87;13 and 95;5. The odds for girls compared to boys of being "at right age" vs the other categories are $(0.55/0.45)/(0.68/0.32) = 0.58$. The odds for "at right age" or "too early" vs "should not have happened" are $(0.87/0.13)/(0.95/0.05) = 0.35$. These are both in the same direction but not particularly close. Based on the discussion in Chapter 6 and the reassurances from the authors of the paper one might be happy that the assumption of proportional odds is met.

Chapter 7

1) Figure 7.3 is a forest plot.
2) It is difficult to tell. The CIs overlap and the lower limit of the six-month interval nearly includes the point interval of the three-month interval, suggesting they are not statistically significantly different.
3) This is because the software used by the authors truncated the results at 0 and 1 respectively if Q is less than its degree of freedom.
4) There is little evidence of heterogeneity at three months, weak evidence at six months, but overall combining three and six months there is clear evidence of heterogeneity.
5) $I^2 = 100(3.61 - 1)/3.61 = 72.3\%$ $H^2 = 3.61/1 = 3.61$.
6) There are three degrees of freedom for Q because there are four studies.

Chapter 8

1) When time = 0 and Region = 0 we have ICCM Speed is 23.8%.
2) January 2019 is 13 months after January 2018, so we would expect $23.8 + 13 \times 0.48 = 29.56\%$.
3) 23.80 + 55.24 = 79.04.
4) A drop of 1.62% when the pandemic was declared.
5) No, it is assumed that the slopes are independent of region.
6) It is not clear, since the authors do not say, but presumably they were not statistically significantly different to region 1. This is not good practice. All coefficients (significant or not) should be given for a model.

Glossary

Analysis of covariance (ANCOVA) A form of linear model with a continuous outcome variable, some categorical input variables and usually just one continuous input variable.

Analysis of variance (ANOVA) A form of linear model with a continuous outcome variable and categorical input variables.

Autoregressive model A model for a time dependent outcome variable in which the error term includes past values of itself.

Bayesian methods Methods which allow parameters to have distributions. Initially the parameter θ is assigned a prior distribution $P(\theta)$, and after data, X, have been collected a posterior distribution $P(\theta|X)$ is obtained using *Bayes' Theorem*, which links the two via the **likelihood** $P(X|\theta)$.

Binary variable A variable which can take only two values, say "success" and "failure".

Binomial distribution The distribution of a **binary variable** when the probability of a "success" is constant.

Bootstrap A computer intensive resampling method to calculate standard errors without relying on model assumptions.

Censored data An observation is censored at X if all we know is that the observation is $\geq X$. Often used with survival data, where all we know is that a subject has survived X amount of time.

Cluster randomised trial A trial in which the subjects are randomised in clusters.

Cochrane–Orcutt method A method of removing **serial correlation** in regression models.

Collider bias A general term which includes Berkson's Bias, where a common cause (i.e. collider) is conditioned in some way that distorts/falsely causes an association between an exposure and disease of interest.

Complementary log-log transform If $0 < P < 1$ then the transform is $\log_e[-\log(1 - P)]$. Used as an alternative to the **logit transform** in **logistic regression**.

Confounder A variable that is related to the exposure and disease of interest, but is not on the causal pathway of the two.

Conditional logistic regression Used to analyse binary data from matched case-control studies, or from cross-over trials.

Statistics at Square Two: Understanding Modern Statistical Application in Medicine, Third Edition.
Michael J. Campbell and Richard M. Jacques.

Continuation ratio model A form of **ordinal regression model**. Suppose we have a three-level ordinal outcome and a binary explanatory variable. If p_1, p_2 and $p_3 = 1 - p_1 - p_2$ are the probabilities of a subject being in levels 1, 2 or 3 when the explanatory variable is at one value and q_1, q_2 and $q_3 = 1 - q_1 - q_2$ are the probabilities of a subject being in levels 1, 2 or 3 when the explanatory variable is the other value. Then the model assumes: $[p_2/(p_1 + p_2)]/[q_2/(q_1 + q_2)] = p_3/q_3$

Design effect (DE) The amount that a variance of an estimator has to be inflated to allow for clustering or other aspects of the sampling scheme.

Deviance A measure of how far a set of data varies from a perfect fit to the data. For Normally distributed residuals it is equal to the residual sum of squares.

Dummy variables Binary variables used for fitting categorical terms, in which each dummy takes the value 0 or 1, and if there are n categories, there are $n - 1$ independent dummy variables.

Durbin–Watson test A test for **serial correlation** in a time series.

Effect modification Given a model with an input variable and an outcome, effect modification occurs if the observed relationship is changed markedly when a third variable is included in the model. An extreme example of this is **Simpson's paradox**.

Extra-Binomial or extra-Poisson variation This occurs when the variation in the data, allowing for the covariates, is greater than would be predicted by the Binomial (or Poisson) distribution.

Fixed effect A term in a model that can be fitted using **dummy variables**. The assumption is that if a new set of data were to be collected, the population parameter would be the same (fixed). Thus the effect of an intervention in a trial is assumed fixed.

Forest plot A plot used in **meta-analysis**. Usually it comprises a series of estimates and confidence intervals from the component studies, and a summary estimate and confidence interval. Supposedly named because it appears like a set of trees.

Funnel plot A plot used in **meta-analysis** to try and detect **publication bias**. It comprises a plot of the precision of estimates of treatment effects from component studies vs the estimate itself.

Generalised estimating equations (gee) A set of equations for estimating parameters in a model, essentially equal to iteratively re-weighted **least squares**. They are commonly used with a **sandwich estimator** to obtain the standard error. There is also **GEE2**, which includes the variance estimators in the set of equations.

Hazard rate The probability per time unit that a case that has survived to the beginning of the respective interval will fail in that interval. Specifically, it is computed as the number of failures per time units in the respective interval, divided by the average number of surviving cases at the mid-point of the interval.

Hazard ratio (Relative hazard) The hazard ratio compares two groups differing in treatments or prognostic variables, etc. If the hazard ratio is 2.0, then the rate of failure in one group is twice the rate in the other group. Can be interpreted as a **relative risk**.

Hierarchical model A model in which factors nest within one another. Thus patients are nested with a doctor who is within a practice. Also known as a **multilevel model**.

Hosmer–Lemeshow statistic A measure of the goodness-of-fit of a **logistic regression** when at least one of the explanatory variables is continuous.

Influential points In regression analysis, points which, if deleted and the model refitted, would have a big effect on at least one of the model parameters.

Intermediary variable An intermediary variable serves as a causal link between other variables. It is acted on by the independent variable and then acts itself on the dependent variable.

Kaplan–Meier plot An empirical plot of the probability of survival on the *y*-axis by survival time on the *x*-axis. Censored observations can be incorporated in the plot.

Latent variables are variables that are not directly observed but are rather inferred through a mathematical model from other variables that are observed (directly measured). Latent variables may correspond to aspects of physical reality. These could in principle be measured, but may not be for practical reasons. In this situation, the term hidden variables is commonly used (reflecting the fact that the variables are meaningful, but not observable). Other latent variables correspond to abstract concepts, such as categories, behavioural or mental states, or data structures. They are used in factor analysis, **random effect models** and **structural equation models**.

Least squares A method of estimating parameters in a model when the outcome is continuous. It fits a linear model by minimising the residual sum of squares. Weighted least squares applies weights to the residuals, usually the inverse of a variance estimate. Iteratively reweighted least squares allows the weights to vary depending on the current fitted values and so requires iteration to be solved.

Leverage points In regression analysis, observations that have an extreme value on one or more explanatory variable. The leverage values indicate whether or not *X* values for a given observation are outlying (far from the main body of the data). They may be **influential points**.

Likelihood The probability of a set of observations given a model. If the model has a single parameter θ, it is denoted $P(X|\theta)$, where *X* denotes the data.

Likelihood ratio test A general purpose test of model M_0 against an alternative M_1 where M_0 is contained within M_1. It is based on the ratio of two likelihood functions one derived from each of H_0 and H_1. The statistics: $-2ln(L_{M0}/L_{M1})$ has approximately a chi-square distribution with d.f. equal to the difference in the number of parameters in the two models.

Linear model A model which is linear in the parameters, but not necessarily in the variables. Thus $y = \beta_0 + \beta_1 X + \beta_2 X^2$ is a linear model but $y = \exp(\beta_0 + \beta_1 X)$ is not.

Logistic regression Used to analyse data where the outcome variable is **binary**. It uses the **logistic** transform of the expected probability of "success".

Logit transform If $0 < P < 1$ then: $\text{logit}(P) = \log_e[P/(1-P)]$. When the outcome is binary, often also called the **logistic** transform.

Maximum likelihood A method of fitting a model by choosing parameters that maximise the **likelihood** of the data.

Meta-analysis A statistical technique used to synthesise results when study effect estimates and their variances are available, yielding a quantitative summary of results.

Mixed model A model that mixes **random** and **fixed effect** terms.

Multiple linear regression Often just known as **multiple regression**. Used to analyse data when the outcome is continuous and the model is **linear**.

Odds If p_1 is the probability of a success, the odds is the ratio of the probability of a success to a failure: $p_1/(1-p_1)$

Odds ratio Used as a summary measure for binary outcomes. If p_1 is the probability of a success in one group and p_2 the probability of success in another, then the odds ratio is: $[p_1/(1-p_1)]/[p_2/(1-p_2)]$

Ordinal regression Used to analyse data when the outcome variable is ordinal. Usually uses the **proportional odds** model or the **continuation ratio** model.

Ordinal variable A categorical variable, where the categories can be ordered, such as pain scores of "mild", "moderate" and "severe".

Over-dispersion In a Poisson and Binomial model, the variance of the outcome is determined by the mean value. When the observed value exceeds this predicted value, the data are said to be over-dispersed. This can happen when the counts are correlated.

Poisson distribution The distribution of a count variable when the probability of an event is constant.

Poisson regression Used to analyse data when the outcome variable is a count.

Prediction Interval Used in Bayesian analysis. A range of values which are a given proportion of the posterior distribution of a parameter.

Propensity score matching This is a statistical matching technique that attempts to estimate the effect of a treatment, policy or other intervention by accounting for the covariates that predict receiving the treatment. It attempts to mimic randomisation and to reduce the bias due to confounding variables that could be found in an estimate of the treatment effect obtained from simply comparing outcomes among units that received the treatment versus those that did not.

Proportional hazards model (*also* the Cox model) Used to analyse survival data. The main assumption is if an explanatory variable is binary, then the **hazard ratio** for this variable is constant over time.

Proportional odds model Used when outcome is ordinal. Suppose we have an ordinal outcome with three categories and a binary explanatory variable. A proportional odds model assumes that the odds ratio for the outcome variable comparing levels 1 and 2 of the outcome is the same as the odds ratio for the outcome variable comparing levels 2 and 3. In the notation used in the definition of the **continuation ratio model** $(p1/(p2+p3))/(q1/(q2+q3) = ((p1+p2)/p_3)/((q_1+q_2)/q_3)$

Publication bias A phenomenon when some studies which have been conducted fail to be published. It usually occurs because studies that have positive findings are more likely to be written up and submitted for publication, and editors are more likely to accept them.

Random effects model A model with more than one random (or error) term. The assumption is that if the study was done again, the terms would estimate different population parameters, in contrast to a **fixed effects** model. Thus in a longitudinal study, the effect of a patient on the outcome is assumed random since a different study would have different patients.

Relative risk Used as a summary measure for binary outcomes for prospective studies. *If* p_1 is the probability of success in one group and p_2 the probability of success in another, the relative risk is p_1/p_2. If p_1 and p_2 are the incidences of an event, then the relative risk is also the **incidence rate ratio**.

Robust standard error (*also* sandwich estimator) A method of estimating standard errors of estimates without assuming the error variances are homogenous.

Sandwich estimator A robust standard error, so-called because the matrix formulation is like a "sandwich" ABA, where A is the "bread" and B the "filling".

Score test A measure of the fit of a set of parameters to a model, based of the slope of the likelihood of the data of model at the null point.

Serial correlation (*also* autocorrelation) In time series when values of a variable are correlated in time.

Simpson's paradox This occurs when one has binary input and output variables and a third variable which is related to both. When a model is fitted that does not include the third variable the observed relationship between the input and output variables is in one direction, and when the third variable is included in the model the direction of the relationship between the input and output variables is reversed.

Stepwise regression Used to decide which of a set of explanatory variables best describes the outcome. Also includes step-up and step-down regression where variables are progressively added or subtracted from the model. It is a purely exploratory technique and should not be used prior to hypothesis testing.

Structural equation modelling This is a statistical technique for testing and estimating causal relations using a combination of statistical data and qualitative causal assumptions. Structural equation modelling may also be explained as a comprehensive statistical approach to testing hypotheses exploring relations between observed and **latent variables.** It is a methodology for representing, estimating and testing a theoretical network of relationships between variables.

Time series regression Regression in which the outcome variable is time dependent.

Wald test A measure of the fit of a parameter of a model based on the estimate of the parameter divided by its estimated standard error.

Weibull distribution A parametric distribution for survival data.

Index

Note: Page numbers followed by "*f*" refer to figures and "*t*" refer to tables.

a

accelerated failure time model 71
alternative hypothesis 141
analysis of covariance (ANCOVA) 18, 20, 25, 31, 52
analysis of variance (ANOVA)
 one-way 30
 repeated measures 83
artificial intelligence 11
autoregressive models 123, 125
autoregressive process 122

b

baseline variable 23, 44
Bayesian approach 85
Bayesian methods 12, 111, 151
 Bayes' theorem 151–152
 computing in 153
 in medical literature 154
 reading and reporting 154
 uses of 152–153
Bayesian statement 146
Bayesian thinking 12
Bayes' theorem 151–152
"bell-shaped" curve 1
Berkson's bias 5
between-doctor variation 80
bias-corrected and accelerated (BCA) method 144
bias-corrected method 144
binary independent variable 42, 65, 102
binary variable 9, 25
Binomial distribution 43, 99
Binomial errors 85
Binomial models 45, 134*f*, 174*t*
 and likelihood 133–135
bootstrap confidence interval for median, 144*t*, 175*t*
bootstrapping and variance robust standard errors 143–144
 example of 144–145
 in medical literature 145–146
 naïve 145
 reporting 149–150
 robust or sandwich estimate SEs 146–147
 robust SEs for unequal variances 147–149
 two-sample t-test with unequal variances 145
 uses of robust regression 149
bootstrap standard error 7
Breslow's method for ties in survival data 69

c

categorical covariates 44
categorical independent variables 22–23, 29–31
causal inference 3–5

Statistics at Square Two: Understanding Modern Statistical Application in Medicine, Third Edition.
Michael J. Campbell and Richard M. Jacques.

causal modelling 12–13
chi-squared distribution 97, 137
cluster randomised trials 81–82, 89
cluster specific model 85
cluster trials 90
Cochrane Collaboration RevMan 113
Cochrane–Orcutt procedure in time series 123, 124*t*, 173, 173*t*
Collider bias 5
competing risks 71–72
complementary log-log plot 72
complex sampling schemes 145
computer-intensive methods 11
conditional logistic regression 58, 60*t*, 166*t*
confidence intervals (CIs) 8, 83, 97, 139, 143
confirmatory analysis 10, 14
confounding 2–3, 51, 52, 102, 121
continuation ratio model 103
continuous independent variables 22, 28
continuous variables 1, 2
Cox model 65, 76
Cox regression model 67–69, 71, 74, 77
cumulative logit model 100
cut points 101

d

data, types of 1–2
degrees of freedom 24
dependent variable 17
design effect (DE) 80
deviance residuals for binary data 140
Direct Acyclic Graph (DAG) 3, 4*f*, 5*f*, 12
discontinuity design 122
discrete quantitative variable 95
Dose Adjustment for Normal Eating (DAFNE) 90
dummy variables 22, 23, 32, 37, 44, 56–58, 62, 81, 84, 97, 113, 124, 126
Durbin–Watson test 123, 126

e

effect modification 2–3
effect modifier 3
Empirical Bayes 153
endogenous variable 12
exchangeable model 80
exploratory analysis 10, 14
exponentials and logarithms 129–131
extra-Binomial variation 45–46, 99
extra-Poisson variation 99

f

fitting models 6–7
fixed effect analysis 57, 84
fixed effect model 81
force of mortality 66
forest plot 111, 112
frailty 81
frequentist approach 12
"fully Bayesian" 153
funnel plot 114, 115*f*, 172*f*

g

generalised estimating equations (gee) 79, 85, 87, 91
"generalised linear models" 6

h

hazard rate 66
hazard ratio 68, 70, 72, 75, 76
hierarchical data structures 80
hierarchical model 81, 153
Hosmer–Lemeshow statistic 53–55
hypothesis testing 7, 137–138

i

incidence rate ratio (IRR) 96, 97
independent variable 12, 17, 25, 27–28, 45
influential point 33, 34, 44, 54
intermediate variable (IM) 4
interrupted time series 122
intra-cluster correlation (ICC) 79, 80

k

Kaplan–Meier
  plots 65, 71, 75
  survival curve 67, 69
  survival plots 69*f*, 167*f*

l

last observation carried forward (LOCF) 11
latent variables 12
least squares, principle of 23, 136
likelihood and gee 85
likelihood ratio (LR) 98, 137–138
linear mixed model 90
"linear models" 5
linear predictor 18
linear regression models 23, 168
lmerTest library 168
logarithms 129–131
logistic or logit transform 43
logistic regression 42, 43, 76, 79, 91, 95, 96, 103
logistic transform 46
logit transform 43
log-linear model 100

m

machine learning 11
Mann–Whitney test 102
marginal model 85
Markov chain Monte Carlo (MCMC) 153
maximum likelihood and significance tests
  binomial models and likelihood 133–135
  confidence intervals (CIs) 139
  deviance residuals for binary data 140
  grouped data 140
  hypothesis testing 137–138
  Normal model 135–137
  Poisson model 135
  score test 138–139
  ungrouped data 140–141
  Wald test 138
maximum likelihood model 86
maximum likelihood random effects models 168, 169*t*
McNemar's chi-square test 58–59
mediation and effect modification 2–3
meta-analysis 107
  examples from medical literature 114–115
  interpreting computer output 113–114
  missing values 111
  models for 108–111
  results
    displaying 111–112
    reading 116
    reporting 115–116
meta-regression 111
missing values 11–12, 111
mixed models 80
model-based approach 12
model fitting and analysis 10
multi-centre trials 83–84
multi-level models 80
multiple imputation 11
multiple linear regression 9, 32
  assumptions underlying models 32–33
  interpreting computer output 23–31
  model 17–18
  model sensitivity 33–35
  one binary and one continuous independent variable 31–32
  results
    reading 36–37
    reporting 36
  stepwise regression 35–36
  two independent variables 18–23
  uses of multiple regression 18
multiple logistic regression
  alternatives to logistic regression 61
  case-control studies 56
  example of conditional logistic regression in medical literature 60
  examples in medical literature 54–56
  interpreting computer output 47–54
  matched case-control study 58–60
  model 5, 42–44
  model checking 44–46
  results
    reading 61–62
    reporting 61
  unmatched case-control study 56–57
  uses of logistic regression 46–47

multiple regression 18, 37, 45
multistage sampling 79
multivariable model 9

n

natural logarithm 130
Negative Binomial regression 46, 81, 99
Newey–West standard error 123
non-inferiority studies 8
non-informative censoring assumption 66
non-Normal distributions 1
non-Normally distributed data 7
non-Normally distributed variables 1
"non-parametric" data 1
Normal distribution 1, 7, 9, 11, 33, 45, 87, 131, 136
Normality assumption 146
Normal model 135–137, 136*f*
null hypothesis 7–9, 138, 140

o

Odds Ratio (OR) 42, 103
one binary independent variable 25, 26–27, 31–32, 47–50
one continuous independent variable 19–21, 31–32
one-way analysis of variance 30, 84
ordinal independent variable 37
ordinal regression 100–101, 102*t*, 171*t*
  interpreting computer output 101–103
  in medical literature 104
  model checking for 103
  results
    reading 104
    reporting 104
ordinal variable 2, 44, 103, 104
ordinary least squares 18
  at group level 84–85
outcome variables 11
over-dispersed models 81
over-dispersion 45, 46, 49, 99

p

"parametric bootstrap" 144
parametric survival models 71
partial likelihood 68
percentile method 144
Placebo group 48
Poisson distribution 96, 99, 105
Poisson regression model 95, 96, 98*t*, 99, 100*t*, 101, 104, 105, 113, 114*t*, 170*t*, 172*t*
  extensions to 99
  interpreting computer output 96–97
  in medical literature 100
  model checking for 97–98
  results
    reading 104
    reporting 104
  used to estimate relative risks 99–100
potential confounding factors 124
Prais–Winsten/Cochrane–Orcutt procedure 122
prediction interval 100, 111–113, 152
propensity score methods 13
proportional hazard model 65 (*see also* Survival analysis)
proportional hazards assumption, 73*t*, 167*t*
proportional odds 100
  assumption 101
  model 101, 103, 104
publication-bias 111, 114

q

qualitative data 1, 2
quantitative data 1

r

random effects models 12, 46, 79–81, 83–85, 91, 99, 112, 113
  cluster randomised trials 81–82
  interpreting computer output 85–87
  logistic regression 85
  in medical literature 90–91
  in meta analysis 110
  model checking 89
  multi-centre trials 83–84
  ordinary least squares at group level 84–85
  random vs fixed effects 81
  repeated measures 82–83

results
reading 90
reporting 89–90
sample surveys 83
random intercepts model 80
"randomised quantile residuals" 45
random vs fixed effects 81
R codes 157–177
regression coefficients 6, 70, 101
regression on group means 169*t*
regression parameters 6
Relative Risk (RR) 5, 41, 70, 96, 99, 108
repeated measures 82
REPOSE cluster randomised controlled trial 90
residuals, leverage and influence 33–34
Restricted (or Residual) Maximum likelihood (REML) 113
robust regression
for unequal variances 148–149*t*, 177*t*
uses of 149
robust standard error (SE) 85, 86, 96, 99, 168*t*
bootstrapping and variance (*see* bootstrapping and variance robust standard errors)

s
sandwich estimator 85, 146, 170
saturated model 98, 134
score test 138–139
semi-parametric models 66
serial correlation 122
significance tests 7
simple cluster trial 82
simple fixed effects model 109
simple random effects model 110
Simpson's paradox 51
"sparse data bias" 55
"sparse data problem" 76
standard errors (SEs) 23, 68, 96, 138, 143
robust or sandwich estimate 146–147
for unequal variances, robust 147–149
standardised mean difference (SMD) 108
standardised mortality ratio (SMR) 96
standardised regression coefficients 31, 34
standardised variables 22
statistical models 5–6
statistical synthesis methods 115
statistical tests using models 8–9
step-down or backwards regression 35
step-up or forwards regression 35
stepwise regression 35–36
stratified Cox model 71 (*see also* survival analysis)
stratified models 70–72
stratified random sampling 145
structural equation model 12
Student's t-test 7
sum of squares (SS) 18
survival analysis 65
example in medical literature 74–76
generalisations of the model 70–72
interpretation of the model 70
interpreting computer output 68–70
model 66–68, 72–73
results
reading 74
reporting 73–74
uses of Cox regression 68

t
"3D plot," for multiple regression 28
time dependent covariates 71
time series regression models 121, 173
estimation using correlated residuals 122–123
interpreting computer output 123
in medical literature 124–125
model 122
results
reading 125
reporting 125
traditional frequentist approach 151
two binary independent variables 51–52
two continuous independent variables 52–54
two independent variables 18–23
two-sample t-test with unequal variances 145

u
"under-dispersion" 46
unequal variances, robust regression for, 148–149*t*, 177*t*
ungrouped data 140–141
uninformative censoring assumption 66
uninformative prior 153

v
variables 9–10

w
Waldlikelihood ratio test 138
Wald test 7, 50, 99, 100, 138, 139
Weibull distribution 71
Winbugs 153
within-doctor variation 80

z
zero-inflated Poisson (ZIP) models 99
z-test 7